AME
HEALTH CARE
ISN'T BROKEN

THE MAXIMIZER'S GUIDE™ TO UNDERSTANDING – VOLUME I

How the American Health Care Cartel
is Undermining American Prosperity

Michael Akinyele

First Edition
Maximizer Media

Copyright © 2021 by Michael Olaoluwa Akinyele. All rights reserved.

Published by Maximizer Media, Upper Marlboro, Maryland

Primal White supremacy, Elitist White supremacy, Benevolent Capitalist, Maximizer Mentality, and Electoral College Per Capita are trademarks of The Maximizer Group, LLC.

The front cover image of rising and descending arrows, the three circles of the root causes below the surface, and the back cover derivative are trademarks of The Maximizer Group, LLC.

Cover design, images, photos, charts, and tables are original, copyrighted works of the author. All rights reserved.

No part of this publication may be reproduced, stored in a retrieval system, or transmitted in any form or by any means, electronic, mechanical, photocopying, recording, scanning, or otherwise without the publisher's prior written permission. Only as permitted under Section 107 or 108 of the 1976 United States Copyright Act.

Interested parties should submit requests to the publisher for permission at https://themaximizergroup.com/about/

Limit of Liability/Disclaimer of Warranty: While the publisher and the author have used their best efforts in preparing this book, they make no representations or warranties concerning the accuracy or completeness of the contents of this book. The advice and strategies contained herein may not be suitable for your situation. You should consult with a professional where appropriate. Neither the publisher nor author shall be liable for any loss of profit or any other commercial damages, including but not limited to special, incidental, consequential, or other damages.

Library of Congress Cataloging-in-Publication Data:

LCCN: 2021910897

ISBN: 978-1-955817-00-4

Second Print: 2021

Maximizer:

A person who consistently seeks the optimal outcome for any endeavor

For Briella, Arielle, and Michelle

"Never apologize for being correct.

Many people, especially ignorant people, want to punish you for speaking the truth, for being correct, for being you.

*Never apologize for being correct
or for being years ahead of your time.*

If you're right and you know it, speak your mind.

Even if you are a minority of one, the truth is still the truth.

– Mahatma Gandhi

Contents

Foreword i

Prologue: We Can Achieve Better Health Outcomes v

Brief Introduction to My Story 1

Two Worlds Collide 25

Summary of My Career Journey 41

Perils of Elevating Mediocrity 55

The American Health Care Ecosystem Isn't Broken 73

Overview of the American Health Care Cartel 95

Physician Burnout 117

Roles and Incentives of Key Stakeholders 131

Key Drivers of High Costs and Health Spending 147

Health Reform 157

Barriers Obstructing Critical Pathways 167

Key Stakeholder Reactions to Reform Efforts 177

Uncompetitive Market Dynamics 187

Non-adherence to Evidence-based Clinical Guidelines............. 197

Potential Solutions 205

Actualizing Paradigm-shifting Change 239

Epilogue: Frustrations 283

Acknowledgments 297

About the Author 303

*"Of all forms of inequality,
injustice in health is most shocking
and the most inhuman
because it often results in physical death."*

– Rev. Dr. Martin Luther King Jr.
Presentation at the Second National Convention
of the Medical Committee for Human Rights, Chicago, 25 March 1966

Foreword

The American health care system, as the title of this book implies, may not be broken. But for many Americans, particularly those from disadvantaged communities and communities of color, it sure isn't working.

Yet, though they bear a disproportionate burden of the dysfunction of the American health care system, the voices heard most loudly in the discussions of health system reform, including mine, often do not come from those communities.

For this reason, this book by Michael Akinyele, an immigrant from Nigeria with a royal lineage, brings a unique insight. Michael has an MBA from Stanford University and an undergraduate degree in Economics from Howard University.

He draws on his experiences consulting for health care companies and leading the innovation center at the U.S. Department of Veterans Affairs (VA).

He does not pull any punches.

There are ideas presented that you will not agree with: that I do not agree with. For example, the chapter on potential solutions critiques many major concepts proposed by many well-known voices (including mine). You (and I) may disagree with Michael's logic that focuses on the reactions of the broad forces that shape health care. But rigorous, dry evaluations of options are not the appeal of the book. The language is intentionally provocative, even inflammatory, and as a result, you may find parts of the narrative offensive (as I do in places).

I believe that all of this is intentional.

If you are expecting a politically correct, analytic assessment of the ills in health care and suggested solutions, this book is not for you. Instead, you will find a critical, personal, and passionate reflection on our health care systems' core problems and aspirational solutions.

Michael's thesis goes well beyond the idea that we need to change consumer and patient incentives to improve competition or that we need to alter how health care providers are paid or how they are organized.

Our problems are more than can be solved by better information technology or artificial intelligence.

Instead, the book's central premise is that the ills of the American health care system reflect the broader ills of American society. It blends economic, sociological, and political viewpoints to argue that the macro structures that are the basis of American society and our health care system work against easy fixes.

More significant changes, reflecting voices across the spectrum, will be needed.

Two quotes embody the themes of this book:

1. Edison's electric light did not come from continuous improvement of the candle. (Oren Harari)
2. In a chronically leaking boat, energy devoted to changing vessels is more productive than energy devoted to patching leaks. (Warren Buffett)

I am not well suited to evaluate the arguments made.

And the appeal for me is as much about the perspective as the substance. But I say with some confidence that this perspective and style is unique.

The narrative jumps from an autobiographical tone, describing the experiences that a well-educated Black man has endured as he strived to achieve the American dream, to a reflective tone remarking on the problems we face to an aspirational discussion of possible solutions.

It draws on events and history well outside of health care, providing a personal interpretation of past events, often in the context of health care.

As a reader, you may infer that Michael is bitter.

I do not believe that this is the case.

Quite contrary, he has a genuine appreciation for both the opportunities he has been afforded in America and for the market-oriented structures that may ultimately provide the disruption he argues is necessary. Yet, he does not shy away from calling out actors and mindsets he views as impeding progress.

MICHAEL CHERNEW, Ph.D.
Chair of the Medicare Payment Advisory Commission (MedPAC)

Prologue:
We Can Achieve Better Health Outcomes

"Never doubt that a small group of thoughtful, committed citizens can change the world. Indeed, it is the only thing that ever has."
– Margaret Mead

This book explores viable approaches to arresting and resolving cancer metastasizing at the intersection of American health care and White supremacy: a calamity that results in pervasive chronic illness, economic malaise, rising rates of diseases and deaths of despair, and avoidable health inequities. This exploration highlights inequities in COVID-19 and maternal mortality outcomes. Inequities between historically marginalized communities and White communities.

Cancer metastasizing at the intersection of American health care and White supremacy is undermining American prosperity. This cancer is curable. In this context, cancer is an evil or destructive practice that is hard to contain or eradicate.

Absent effective intervention, this cancer will continue to ravage the host.

It may kill the host.

Cancers are deadly. Excruciating. Debilitating.

Often incurable. Sometimes fatal.

We've all lost people we know, or care about, to cancer.

I have.

We are losing people we know, or care about, to cancer.

I am.

We will lose people we know, or care about, to cancer.

Unless we intervene, arrest, and resolve cancer before it metastasizes.

We must be willing to do whatever it takes after cancer metastasizes.

We must fight the urge to feel helpless. Hopeless. Fatalistic.

I am building a coalition of change agents—also known as maximizers—and justice activists who are similarly appalled by how the racial hierarchy propagated by White supremacy informs the American health care ecosystem to the detriment of society and equitable economic growth. The calamity manifesting at the intersection of White supremacy and American health care enables evil outcomes and looming economic destruction.

The complexities of White supremacy make it difficult to comprehend; this, in turn, makes it easy for many individuals and organizations to deny perpetuating it within their daily practices.

Many deny upholding White supremacy.

For the themes highlighted within this book, White supremacy is boiled down to an evil mindset that embraces the belief that access to economic opportunity and positions of authority should first or solely be provided to White males ahead of more capable males of color or females of any race.

Although this evil mindset is pervasive across American society, many individuals, organizations, and institutions are quick to denounce White supremacy when racial tensions flare up. The rhetoric is particularly elevated during periods of civil unrest that typically follow publicized incidents of racial discrimination and state-sponsored violence against people of color.

While the rhetoric is loud during periods of civil unrest, I refuse to get distracted. Instead, I focus on actions pursued and outcomes achieved by individuals, organizations, and institutions who claim not to be upholders of White supremacy. As the Bible says in the book of Matthew chapter 7 verse 16, "by their fruits, you shall know them."

White supremacy enables the advancement of mediocre White males over more capable males of color and females of any race. This disparity is evident when evaluating the criteria used by institutions and organizations to elevate White males to positions of authority and simultaneously overlook qualified males of color and females of any race. A reality manifested in the disparities in representation of White males to males of color and females of any race who are in positions of authority in institutions and organizations that enable this evil mindset.

This book attempts to simply boil White supremacy down to a narrow and relatively easy construct to comprehend. However, its use in this book is broadly synonymous with systemic racism.

Systemic racism manifests as policies and practices throughout a society or organization that grant race-based unfair favoritism to people of a certain race. Usually, persons from the dominant race are favored. That same system levies an unjust or harmful prejudice against other groups of people. Usually, persons from non-dominant races are disfavored.

The cancer of White supremacy manifests in both primal and elitist contexts.

In the primal context, it traumatizes the bodies of those it oppresses.

In the elitist context, it traumatizes their minds.

In exploring the calamity at the intersection of White supremacy and American health care, this book highlights similarities between the racial and oppressive hierarchy propagated by the institution of White supremacy and other institutions that enable the similarly harmful outcomes that result, including the traumatization of those placed at the bottom of those hierarchies.

In evaluating the impact of White supremacy, this book explores the trauma that similarly oppressive hierarchal institutions like patriarchy, polygamy, colorism, European imperialism, and the Nigerian oligarchy have caused across generations. I also share perspectives on the aforementioned oppressive hierarchies through the lens of my personal and professional experiences, human stories, and data. With the different perspectives shared, this book reiterates its central argument.

<u>Established institutions function as designed</u>. They aren't broken or in need of repair.

Americans should reimagine and replace Institutions that yield evil outcomes with a better model or design. To realize the health and life outcomes we seek, we must redesign our institutions to serve everyone they are supposed to serve equitably—<u>We the People</u>.

This book posits that Americans must first acknowledge that the current design of our health care ecosystem doesn't meet the needs of all Americans. We must accept this truth to actualize a simple, affordable, and equitable health care ecosystem.

Subsequently, Americans must pursue the significant redesign required to establish an American health care ecosystem that works for all the beneficiaries it is supposed to serve—<u>We the People</u> of these United States.

I'll be the first to acknowledge that for us to weather the challenges caused by the COVID-19 pandemic, we must increase our investment in the current American health care ecosystem. However, we shouldn't lose sight of the enduring fiscal and societal harms the complex, expensive, and inequitable American health care ecosystem is causing.

Later on in this book, after exploring American health care and the ways its design enables the current malaise, this book also examines tactics commonly utilized by stakeholders to ensure their success. Tactics explored include: Supporting the election of legislators sympathetic to stakeholder viewpoints, gaining the upper hand by hiring influential public servants and career civil servants responsible for implementing or enforcing regulations. And other untoward actions.

Although chapters of this book are devoted to exploring potential solutions that may bring about meaningful change, I recognize and admit that many American health care ecosystem stakeholders seek to maintain the status quo. When compelled to take action, those stakeholders prefer to pursue low-value incremental change.

Those stakeholders are formidable opponents.

They remain undefeated after several attempts at health reform.

The potential solutions examined in this book include some I developed throughout my career. Policies advanced by the Trump Administration. Health care proposals by the Biden-Sanders unity task force team. And recommendations from health reform luminaries featured on the 1% Steps for Health Care Reform website. For the potential solutions explored in this book, I also discuss several scenarios that would neutralize or reverse any beneficial gains achieved even if implementing the recommended solutions goes according to plan.

While I remain hopeful that one day change may come, I recognize that individuals and institutions capable of enabling better outcomes have no incentive to do so. Those individuals and institutions lack the political will to pursue or implement paradigm-shifting ideas.

The final chapter of this book intends to activate enlightened readers to join a coalition of empowered American maximizers and justice activists that are encouraged to fulfill their role in enabling a significant redesign of the American health care ecosystem. A redesign that should yield a virtual-first, consumer-centric American health care ecosystem that is simple, affordable, and equitable.

Although the path is narrow, victory is possible.

To win, Americans must establish a pro-democracy nation.

A nation that can maximize the potential of its population.

A nation capable of enacting the will of the people.

A nation capable of accepting the truth as true.

What is true is always true.

The truth is true. Always.

Lies aren't true.

Alternative facts aren't true.

Unscientific opinions aren't true.

Many scientific facts aren't true.

The Multiregional theory was a scientific theory opposing the scientific views about the Out of Africa Model. Genetic evidence eventually disproved the Multiregional theory. According to Multiregional theory, the ancestors of prehistoric homosapiens left Africa 2 million years ago. Not true. They settled in different places around the world. Not true. They evolved to humans in Europe and Asia. Not true.

There is more genetic variation between different groups of some modern-day Africans than the genetic differences found in some modern-day Africans and Eurasians. That's the truth.

The prevailing scientific fact is that the ancestors of prehistoric homosapiens evolved into humans on the African continent. 200,000 years ago. Not 2 million. They lived on the continent for over 100,000 years before strategically migrating to different parts of the world. Less than 70,000 years ago.

We are all members of the human race, initially sourced from the same place.

We are stronger together.

Artificially divided. Decaying.

Our health is our wealth.

We are not healthy.

Wealthy, we are not.

We can only avoid the economic destruction and erosion of consumer value expected to occur across future

American health care markets if we implement meaningful reforms to campaign finance corruption, partisan gerrymandering, and voter suppression laws. Unless there are significant gains on those three fronts, <u>all attempts</u> to evolve American health care into a simple, affordable, and equitable health care ecosystem <u>will fail</u>.

I hope all who read this book are empowered to actualize a reduction in the confusion and stress enabled by the complexity, high prices, and inequities of the American health care ecosystem. While it might be comforting to view ignorance as bliss, when interacting with American health care, preparation and knowledge are vital to avoiding devastating outcomes associated with engaging the American health care ecosystem from a position of ignorance.

I'm grateful for the hundreds of health care industry experts, consumers, regulators, executives, and investors I've had the pleasure of engaging with over the last couple of years while evaluating the future of value-based care and payment innovation. Given my overall alignment with frustrations and perspectives shared, I was finally inspired to write and publish this book.

While I wrote the outline for the majority of this book in 2017, I felt compelled to put pen to paper in this pivotal moment. Inspired by the phrase invented by Sir Edward Bulwer-Lytton, "the pen is mightier than the sword." The world is still contending with the global COVID-19 pandemic that continues to decimate primarily Black and Brown households.

Tomorrow is not guaranteed. My lived experiences uniquely qualify me to share uncommon insights about the American health care ecosystem's current design and inner workings. We recently lost Black male icons in their prime. Kobe Bryant. Chadwick Boseman. If the "universe" can take them out, what hope do I, a regular Black man, have?

I also don't want to be overly optimistic and assume I will be alive long enough to personally explain to my children the insights I share in this book. I've often contemplated creating content—recording videos and writing manuscripts of my musings and principles—that can be shared with my children if I die before they reach adulthood.

However, I've had a lot more fun incorporating those musings, principles, and lived experiences into this book. I would also like to think that memorializing my perspectives in published content can be more impactful.

Finally, to better prepare my children to succeed in this world that my wife and I invited them to, I think it's important they learn the value of developing unique perspectives and summoning the courage to share those perspectives with the world. It would be beneficial for them to learn from my example.

I was born in Nigeria and immigrated to the United States in 2002.

I became a naturalized citizen in 2011.

As I celebrate my 10th year as an American citizen, I'm still coming to terms with my evolving relationship with this great nation I'm privileged to call home.

Often oscillating between feelings of gratitude, fear, hope, and despair, I remain appreciative of the accomplishments I've been privileged to achieve while living in America. Though eternally grateful, I remain burdened by the impact that White supremacy has on life in America. On life around the world.

My children were born in America and can run for President If they want to. I hope and pray my wife and me and our extended families can raise them to be capable, benevolent, and self-assured adults poised to help make our nation and the world a better place.

Special thanks to my wife and children. They are my legacy and most valuable assets☺. Thanks for putting up with my quirks. Many thanks to my parents, siblings, extended family, church family, and mentors who raised me and helped shape my perspective and outlook on life.

I'm also thankful for all the organizations that accepted or rejected me over the years. The countless encounters—positive and negative—catalyzed by our interactions helped make me who I am today.

I wrote this book to hopefully provide clarity, illumination, and a viable approach to resolving cancer metastasizing at the intersection of White supremacy and American health care.

I hope all who read this book and are inspired to act, think boldly and execute pragmatically. I hope inspired persons focus on solving significant pain points while maximizing opportunities to pursue paradigm-shifting reform of the American health care ecosystem.

Despite my predominantly pessimistic overtones, I have faith in humanity and believe that the power to enable a better future is within each of us.

There's no time like the present to invent the future we seek.

We just have to muster the courage to do the right thing.

"Truth sounds like hate to those who hate truth."
— Dr. George C. Fraser

Brief Introduction to My Story

"The unhealthy gap between what we preach in America and what we often practice creates a moral dry rot that eats at the very foundation of our democratic ideals and values." – Whitney M. Young

B eing a Black man in America is the single greatest <u>trauma</u>-inducing reality of my existence.

<u>Trauma</u> I remain hopeful I can help my children cope with as they grow up in America.

<u>Trauma</u> I wish my children won't have to deal with as they are trying to build a life in a country and world where they are likely to be perceived as less than, unintelligent, and dangerous, simply because of the color of their skin.

I remain <u>traumatized</u> by my personal experiences with racism.

I am <u>traumatized</u> by the publicized murders of Black people by state-sanctioned authorities like the police.

I am <u>traumatized</u> by White "dudes" or "dudettes" who remain emboldened to weaponize race to destroy or curtail Black life while shrinking access to economic opportunities for Black people.

"Dudes" or "dudettes" are separate and distinct from men or women with evolved mindsets. Real men and women reject delusional thinking and recognize the harms of rudimentary mindsets rooted in racism, bigotry, misogyny, and patriarchy.

While I've experienced several unpleasant interactions with the police and remain grateful that I drove or walked away physically unharmed, I remain <u>traumatized</u>. The pain and

<u>trauma</u> of the unnecessary humiliation associated with most of those encounters continue to haunt me.

Although I can reasonably predict and avoid social interactions that are likely to expose me to overt racism, it has become increasingly challenging to predict which social interactions will be laced with irritating racial microaggressions.

Over the years, I've gradually withdrawn from most social interactions.

Since the COVID-19 pandemic began, my external, in-person social interactions have essentially dwindled to zero.

Unlike social interactions, academic and professional settings where I am required to engage others have been unavoidable environments. I am engaging others to build my credentials and earn a living. Those same academic and professional situations are where I've experienced some of my most traumatizing and lingering encounters with discrimination.

Even when there is evidence to the contrary, White people are primarily given the benefit of the doubt over Black people. I reached that conclusion after countless interactions with subordinates, peers, and supervisors.

To have a fighting chance, I eventually became adept at documenting evidence and bringing it to light in defense of my dignity, integrity, and forward progression.

Particularly challenging has been my interactions with White "dudettes."

Operating like wolves in sheep's clothing, some White "dudettes" are skilled at presenting themselves as White supremacists in "White ally" clothing. The White terror they are uniquely positioned to unleash is typically activated by "clutching of pearls," "signals of a damsel in distress," and unfounded claims of "intimidation."

Fortunately, my university education primarily transpired at Howard University. An admired Historically Black

College and University (HBCU). I mainly built my career in management consulting. When exposure to toxicity in a particular professional environment pushed me to the brink, working in management consulting enabled me to transition to other projects or lateral to other firms

I went into academic and professional situations prepared to work twice as hard.

<u>Prepared</u> to be allocated inadequate resources.

<u>Prepared</u> to contend with implicit or explicit denigration of my intellect.

<u>Prepared</u> to be unjustifiably labeled intimidating.

<u>Prepared</u> to be expected to "perform miracles."

Despite all my preparation, I was sometimes <u>still unprepared</u> for some of the tactics used to weaponize race to curtail or eliminate my advancement opportunities.

My travels have led me to other countries in different parts of the world. Countries mainly in Africa, Europe, Asia, South America, and the Caribbean—technically just Antigua where my mother-in-law, Barbara, was born and raised. My travels constantly remind me of global anti-Black sentiment, xenophobia, and colorism.

Leisure travel is when the most irritating occurrences—typically racial micro-aggressions—catch me by surprise. The hardest-hitting blows are the ones you don't see coming.

The most recent example transpired during a romantic getaway my wife, Bolanle, and I took to Capetown, South Africa, in 2019. At the end of a night-out in an upscale section of the Victoria and Alfred (V&A) waterfront, a European White "dude" kept insisting I was the hotel shuttle bus driver.

He proceeded to instruct me to bring the bus back to the V&A waterfront mall.

He instructed me to pick him up.

The incident occurred while we were out with another Black couple attending the same marriage retreat that our church organized. Bolanle was visibly pregnant with our youngest, Michelle.

I decided to be on my best behavior.

The second time the European White "dude" came up to the passenger-side to instruct me, I had to irritably explain to him that I wasn't the driver. I explained to him that I was clearly sitting in the passenger's seat with no steering wheel in front of me. There was an awkward, tense silence on the bus as we rode back to the hotel. It was a 20-seater with mostly White tourists.

As we approached the hotel, a pair of European White "dudettes" who sat in the row behind me decided to weigh in––likely motivated by White guilt—by stating, "You shouldn't feel bad. You look responsible, which is why he assumed you were the shuttle bus driver."

I was taken aback by the fact that they had the nerve to try and defend his behavior.

I was further incensed that they had the audacity to state their misguided opinion confidently.

I guess in their collective minds, the purpose of a younger-looking Black man in the upscale V&A waterfront area was either to serve White tourists or to rob them. Given their misguided, racist logic, I guess I should be "grateful" that my presence was assumed to be of service. And not criminal mischief.

I turned around to identify the source of the comment precisely. I noticed Bolanle giving me "the look" as they shared their opinion. I scowled at them disapprovingly and didn't verbally respond to their comment. During and immediately after the incident, I was visibly irritated.

The reality sunk in that even while vacationing on the African continent, I couldn't escape the global reach of White supremacy.

I was born and raised in Ibadan, Oyo State, Nigeria. A country with hundreds of ethnic factions. A country consumed by extreme tribalism and widespread hate and mistrust of the "other." I learned growing up that groups embrace the familiar and fear the "other whenever there is resource scarcity or strife." And instead of the different disadvantaged factions banding together to fight for a better future for all, disadvantaged factions focus on attacking each other.

Disadvantaged factions fight over crumbs from the proverbial "national cake."

Crumbs that dominant groups allow them to have.

Disadvantaged people are the proverbial "masses."

Dominant groups condition the masses to arrive at this outcome by design.

Dominant groups incentivize the masses to retreat into their respective tribal and religious corners, where they can continue to clash and live in squalor. While they fight and live in squalor, dominant groups continue to oppress and exploit the artificially divided masses.

The Marxist view on religion references this phenomenon by espousing the notion that religion is the opiate of the masses. The word opiate is apt because the masses are usually intoxicated by their delusional embrace of fanatical religious beliefs.

Too intoxicated to recognize they are being conditioned.

Bamboozled into acting against their self-interest.

I became aware of the Marxist view on religion after hearing my father reference the phrase mentioned above while lamenting the Nigerian condition. A country like Nigeria manifests the Marxist theory on religion since religious and tribal clashes continue to undermine peace and prosperity. Meanwhile, the oligarchs continue to gobble up chunks of the national cake.

The Marxist view illuminates a Nigerian condition where religion is big business and crooners like Adekunle Gold flood the airways with popular songs like "Pick Up." A song mainly about a protagonist waiting for God to answer his prayer and make him as rich as Aliko Dangote—the wealthiest Black person in the world. A Nigerian man.

Thankfully, there are nascent signs that the Nigerian masses are starting to see through the fog of the ubiquitous "prosperity hustle" in Nigeria.

Examples of such nascent signs became apparent in a Twitter exchange I came across when Elon Musk briefly became the wealthiest person in the world. @OgbeniDipo (Dr. Dipo Awojide) tweeted, "The God that did it for Elon Musk will do it for us." @rsvptemple (Ozioma Temple Egemasi III) replied, "Elon Musk is an Atheist."

Although White supremacy is uniquely dehumanizing and globally pervasive, American institutions that promote White supremacy aren't too dissimilar from institutions in other countries that advantage dominant groups at the expense of other members of society.

As a young child, whenever the topic of "ethnic inequality" in Nigeria was discussed, my paternal grandfather, Chief Michael Okunola Taiwo Akinyele (Chief Akinyele), who bestowed his first name on me, would say, *"Ìka ò dógba."*

Ìka ò dógba is a Yoruba phrase that translates to "fingers are not equal."

I recall inferring from his comment that equality was unachievable and unnecessary for societies to flourish. I assumed such a phrase was easy for him to say since, as an older, Christian, Yoruba male with influence in the Yoruba monarchy and among the educated elite, he enjoyed life at the top of the food chain.

He lived his best life after Nigeria secured its independence from the British Empire.

He was benefiting from all Nigerian society had to offer.

I matured.

I gained clarity from my father on the true meaning of the phrase *"ìka ò dógba."*

I learned the most appropriate inference one should make.

"Everyone has different capabilities."

During periods of sibling rivalry or familial discord, my father would often explain that our family—or any group seeking the same outcome—was stronger together. He would reassure us that even though we were of different ages, genders, and sizes, we all had diverse capabilities that added value to our family unit. As he spoke, he would typically use a balled-up fist to represent the impact we could have as a coordinated unit. In practical terms, he was also illustrating to us that one could do more damage to the opposition with a punch than an open-handed slap.

As an adult, I researched the use of the phrase *"ìka ò dógba"* and the historical context surrounding its use. I discovered alternative inferences like: it is suitable for prosperous members of a group to share their gains with less successful members who can't advance as far.

Even though I initially internalized an interpretation of the phrase *"ìka ò dógba"* that implicitly endorsed societal inequities, I realized that a hand with extreme disparities in finger lengths couldn't be considered "flourishing."

Chief Akinyele retired as a Judge of the Customary Court System of Akinyele Local Government Area (LGA) in Ibadan.

He benefited from his older brothers serving as Officers of the British Empire (OBE).

He benefited from one of his brothers ascending to the throne.

Ọba Isaac Babalola Akinyele (King Akinyele), the Olubadan (King of Ibadan). King Akinyele served as a Knight of the British Empire (KBE). Queen Elizabeth II knighted him during her state visit to Nigeria in 1956.

To strengthen family ties and further share the privilege he enjoyed, King Akinyele named my father and bestowed his first name, Isaac, on my father.

Chief Akinyele named me and bestowed his first name on me. He bestowed my father's second name, Olaoluwa, on me. Growing up, I believed I benefitted from additional privileges because I bore my father and grandfathers' names.

At the time of Nigeria's independence in 1960, Ibadan was the country's largest and most populous city. Ibadan was the second-most populous city in Africa, behind Cairo, Egypt. During British colonial rule, Ibadan was the center of administration of the old Western Region.

The old Western Region was a landmass that consists of present-day Delta, Edo, Ekiti, Kwara, Lagos, Ogun, Ondo, Osun, and Oyo States. The old Western Region was approximately an eighth of the total landmass of Nigeria.

My paternal great-grandfather Josiah Akinyele was our family patriarch. He was the first son of Bolude, a pagan warrior and herbalist from Ibadan. My paternal great-grandfather converted to Christianity in the 1850s and changed his first name from Akinyele to Josiah.

After being baptized, he adopted the former, Akinyele, as his last name.

Many warrior families across Yorubaland—a nation-state that covered a landmass the size of Greece and spanned modern-day Nigeria, Togo, and the Republic of Benin—converted to Christianity.

They subsequently withdrew from their militant ways. Their withdrawal from their militant ways served the European agenda. It helped enable the expansion of European influence in the region. It led to the eventual colonization of Nigeria by the British Empire.

In 1914, Lord Lugard merged the Northern Nigeria Protectorate with the Colony and Protectorate of Southern Nigeria.

The merger served the British Empire well but established a dysfunctional design that still undermines Nigerian prosperity.

Conversion to Christianity also meant a rejection of traditional Yoruba religions, which serves as the basis for present-day religions like *Santería*. When the Church imposed Christianity on the Nordic region around the 900s, they forced the Vikings to abandon pagan gods like Thor—the god of thunder who wields a battle-hammer charged with lightning.

Similarly, the British Empire forced Yorubaland to discard Yoruba deities like *Ṣàngó*—the god of thunder who wields a battle-ax charged with lightning. Setting aside the similarities in Nordic and Yoruba pagan gods, it is evident that the colonialization and subjugation playbook has been in rotation for centuries. One can only hope that humanity would catch a clue at some point and chart a better path forward.

Chief Akinyele was appointed the *Baálẹ̀* of Akinyele. He was the Lord of the landmass that is present-day Akinyele and Ido LGAs. Akinyele was approximately the size of the landmass of the Turks and Caicos Islands. Chief Akinyele was appointed the *Baálẹ̀* mainly because his grandfather, Bolude, owned most of the land, ultimately divided among his many children, and later sold. The people who worked and lived in Akinyele owed tributes to the *Baálẹ̀*.

Fortunately for the masses, Chief Akinyele had a benevolent nature. Also, because of his Christian beliefs, he rejected tributes owed to the *Baálẹ̀*.

In addition to privileges enjoyed by members of the royal elite, as Christians, our family also benefited from being members of the religious elite.

Those benefits grew as the Church became more powerful in Ibadan.

My grandfather's eldest brother, Bishop Alexander Babatunde Akinyele (Bishop Akinyele), was appointed the first Anglican Diocesan Bishop of Ibadan. His brother, King Akinyele, was also a religious leader in his own right. He aligned his section of the Aladura movement with the British Apostolic Church in 1931. He eventually broke away and founded the Christ Apostolic Church (CAC), where he served as President from 1936 till he died in 1964. My father, Isaac, remained a faithful and active CAC member his entire life. He eventually became an Elder at the worldwide CAC Missionary Headquarters at Ita-Baale Olugbode in Ibadan.

Our family also enjoyed the privilege of being members of the educated elite. The Akinyele brothers served as shining examples for Yorubaland. Bishop Akinyele became the first indigene of Ibadan to obtain a university degree after earning a bachelor's degree from Fourah Bay College in 1912. He later founded Ibadan Grammar School, the first secondary school established in Ibadan.

My maternal grandfather, Pa John Alamu Tella (Pa Tella), was a wealthy trader and polygamist from Ejigbo, Osun State, Nigeria. Ejigbo is one of the oldest Yoruba towns and is as ancient as Old Oyo.

Òrànmíyàn, the Prince of Ilé ifè and eventual King of Yorubaland founded Old Oyo. Òrànmíyàn was Odùduwà's youngest son. Odùduwà was a "divine" Yoruba king and the first Òòni (ruler) of Ilé ifè—the Yoruba holy city. Old Oyo was established in the 1300s, and Òrànmíyàn went on to serve as the first Aláàfin of Oyo and concurrently as Oba of Benin.

Pa Tella converted to Christianity in the 1940s after marrying his fifth wife, my maternal grandmother, Madam Mary Adebola Tella (Madam Tella).

He started his career as an elementary school teacher before venturing into the sales and trading business. He initially traded European merchandise like cement, iron, and kerosene but eventually focused his business on trading commodities like cocoa and palm kernel at scale. With the growth of his business, he amassed wealth which he used to acquire assets, including real estate, large swaths of undeveloped land, and a fleet of trucks he used in his trading business.

He donated a portion of his land to the Idi-Ape Baptist Church in Ejigbo. I visited the church for the first time in 2007 during Madam Tella's funeral service. Madam Tella holds a special place in my heart as I did in hers while she was alive. Given the often oppressive hierarchal nature of polygamous families, Madam Tella endured significant mistreatment from the "elder wives."

Madam Tella suffered through the horror of witnessing the premature live burial of her 11-month old son, my uncle. He was coincidentally also named Olaoluwa.

My uncle got infected with smallpox after my mother survived her third bout of the disease. While Madam Tella was tending to him, he started convulsing. Some Black "dudes" in the extended family, likely operating at the behest of the first elder wife—the mother of the only surviving male child sired by Pa Tella—declared my uncle dead.

He was still breathing.

They insisted on burying him immediately.

He was still breathing.

Madam Tella was powerless to stop the Black "dudes" who ripped him out of her hands.

He was still breathing.

They rushed off to bury the 11-month old infant.

He was still breathing.

They buried him.

He was still breathing.

Devastated and traumatized by the event, she grieved his death for decades.

Except for the son born to Pa Tella by his first wife, all his other male children—four in total, including my uncle—died under mysterious circumstances. Those deaths occurred in their infancy, primarily right after they were born.

Unfortunately for the first wife, despite all her scheming, Pa Tella died without a will. The entire extended Tella family got in the fray after Pa Tella's death. They have been squabbling and taking each other to court in the 50-years since Pa Tella passed away. While much of Pa Tella's assets have sold over the years, a material portion remains tied up in legal proceedings.

My mother, Ayoni, the second daughter of Madam Tella—the fifth wife in the Tella compound—also endured mistreatment growing up. The first wife viewed investment in her education as a waste of the family's resources. Thankfully my mother was permitted to attend an elite Catholic secondary school in Kaduna State, Nigeria.

However, after she graduated and gained admission to pursue her bachelor's degree at the University of Ibadan, the first wife refused to approve funding to pay for her fees to attend university. Ironically, the cost of attending her elite secondary school was higher than the projected cost of attending university.

While the first wife rejected my mother's funding request, she told my mother that no other child of Pa Tella had gone to university, so why should she? In a mocking tone, she told my mother that she would eventually end up in someone's kitchen irrespective of whatever academic heights she attains. She will ultimately spend most of her time devoted to domestic household matters.

Fortunately, my mother was able to secure her first-year tuition from an extended family member. After she arrived on campus at the University of Ibadan, she received a full-ride, merit scholarship covering all expenses required for the entire four-year bachelor's degree.

When she went back home during the holidays, she refunded the first-year tuition money she had collected from her extended family member.

My mother was the only female child—out of 10—of Pa Tella to earn a university degree.

After graduating from the University of Ibadan—established in 1948 as the University College London, Ibadan—, she obtained her master's degree in agricultural biochemistry at the University College Wales, Aberystwyth—presently known as Aberystwyth University. She returned to the University of Ibadan to complete her doctoral degree in chemistry.

She started her career as a Chemistry Professor at The Polytechnic, Ibadan.

She retired in 2017 as a chemistry professor—technically a master instructor—at Howard University.

As I grew up in Ibadan, I came to appreciate and leverage all the privileges I enjoyed as a Black, Christian, and Yoruba male descended from reputable Yoruba families in South-West Nigeria. Yoruba culture and people are dominant in southwestern Nigeria. I carried myself with confidence and a tinge of arrogance. My confidence was rooted in a mindset that I could achieve anything I wanted if I stayed in God's will. The tinge of arrogance was rooted in the legacy of my forefathers' achievements.

Knowledge of my family's accomplishments instilled in me a strong sense of self-worth and cemented the belief that I could be as good as anyone else.

Unfortunately, some of that strong sense of self-worth manifested as entitlement, which is frowned upon in Yoruba culture. Being entitled is viewed as particularly offensive when coming from a younger person.

Some of my earliest memories are of my parents chastising me for being rude or disrespectful to elders, reminding me to be humble while saying, *"ránti ọmọ ẹni tí ìwọ n ṣe."* A Yoruba phrase that translates to "remember whose child you are."

While I'm sure my parents intended for the statement to remind me always to pursue excellence and bring honor to the family, it often just fanned the flames of my overinflated ego. It caused me to nurture my inner "douchebag."

Some of my proudest moments came when I enrolled in any new class and attendance was taken. My new teachers would often ask if I was related to my father or family. A big smile would sprout on my face, and I would proudly proclaim, yes, I am!

Outside of the classroom setting, I usually remembered the phrase when school bullies challenged me or traffic police stopped me—after I started driving. I would usually direct my ire at the offending party by boldly stating, "Do you know who my father is?" In many instances, I would usually go on to reference my family name or my father on earth, proudly declaring that "I'm the son of Professor Olaoluwa Akinyele."

Like my father, I primarily used my Yoruba name, Olaoluwa, when I lived in Nigeria.

I would also channel my father in heaven. Mostly inaudibly or in my head.

When occasion demanded, I proudly proclaimed, "I am a child of the most-high God."

Given the pervasive paternalistic culture in Nigeria and ubiquitous familial ties to royalty, most Nigerian-born males, especially Yoruba ones, presume they are special—god's "gift" to women—, develop an inflated sense of self and a god complex—I'm generalizing.

The worst offenders earned the moniker "Yoruba Demon" for their philandering ways, conquests, and exploits.

Like many Yoruba males, growing up, I was afflicted with an inflated sense of self and a god complex. I still exhibit some of those tendencies today, which is one reason I think I'm a bit of an acquired taste and typically only get along with self-assured people. Exacerbating those tendencies are some Obsessive-Compulsive Personality Disorder (OCPD) traits I occasionally exhibit.

Growing up in Ibadan, I lived a sheltered life because my parents instituted household rules that restricted our interaction with "outsiders" to the times we were in school or church. While I considered most household rules irritating, I no longer fault my parents for their approach. I now recognize they likely suffered from elevated paranoia developed from traumatic events they experienced growing up.

My mother, in an oppressive polygamous compound.

The Olubadan's palace exposed my father to the inner workings of the Yoruba monarchy.

Living in the Olubadan's palace exposed him to several failed attempts to assassinate his uncle, King Akinyele.

A palace where he once witnessed his father, Chief Akinyele, wrestle and disarm an assailant trying to stab the King.

Due to the restrictions on our interaction with outsiders, my siblings and I spent most of our free time indoors, mostly consuming Hollywood, Bollywood, and Nollywood content. Fortunately, I am acutely aware of my ancestors' accomplishments and didn't internalize any propaganda baked into the foreign content.

I was exposed to the "White savior" propaganda hardwired into most American movies like Star Wars, Green Mile, and Dangerous Minds.

I was also exposed to "family-friendly" manifestations of propaganda embedded into sitcoms like Different Strokes and Webster. I didn't buy into what they were selling.

Growing up, I benefited from being aware of my ancestors' accomplishments and social status, their privileged membership within the ruling aristocracies of Yorubaland, and the historical occurrence of African reverse colorism that manifested as violence and discrimination against albinos.

The historical African oppression of albinos caused some families to abandon their newly born children afflicted with albinism.

The worst manifestation of the anti-albinism violence was the kidnapping and ritual murder of albinos in different countries across Africa.

While attending primary school, I witnessed my albino classmates suffer from sensitivity to sunlight while enduring taunts from classmates about their "strange Whiteness."

I admired "Whiteness" even less.

I also encountered refugee children from Niger—a nation along the northern border of Nigeria. They solicited alms and pressed their faces against the window of our car whenever we ventured out of the gated campus of the University of Ibadan, the place we called home. The refugee children from Niger had light skin and European features like narrow noses and straight hair.

I admired "Whiteness" even less.

It was relatively easy for me to disregard any propaganda that promoted the message that people with "White skin" are inherently superior. I was aware of my ancestors' accomplishments, historical African issues with albinism, and the plight of the refugees I'd encountered,

On the contrary, I often extrapolated that ancient Africans probably oppressed people with "White skin" the same way some Modern-Era Africans oppressed albinos.

I grew up assuming that ancient Africans drove ancient people with "White skin" out of Africa to less fertile grounds in the deserts and mountains of other continents.

I admired "Whiteness" even less.

And as a child, on a biological level, I just couldn't fathom how "White skin" that is more sensitive to the sun—the source of life/ photosynthesis—, could be inherently superior.

I admired "Whiteness" even less.

With my experiences growing up privileged in Nigeria and awareness of past atrocities committed by Africans against albinos, I believe dominant groups of any race or creed can cause the inexplicable mistreatment of non-dominant members of their respective societies.

Ever since my wife and I got married and started talking about having children, we've been concerned about how and when we would explain racial injustice to our children.

We're still unsure of the timing of the detailed racial justice conversation.

In the interim, we've been doing everything within our power to expose our children to Black excellence. We also reinforce their capabilities and sense of self-worth whenever we can.

Unfortunately, despite our best efforts to bestow our children the solid and proud sense of Black identity and self-worth we grew up with, we're yet to accomplish that goal fully. I was confronted with that gut-wrenching reality when I recently overheard a conversation between our 5-year old, Briella, and her 3-year old sister, Arielle.

Briella explained to Arielle—who has a slightly darker skin tone—that while she was "White," Arielle was "Black." Mortified by the conversation transpiring between the two, I quickly interjected while Arielle looked crestfallen.

I asked Briella why she thought she was White.

She replied, "I don't want to be Black because I don't want to sit in the back of the bus."

I was slightly relieved because it appeared that her comments stemmed from her exposure to the story of Rosa Parks.

I was relieved I didn't have to deconstruct racial injustice to a pair of toddlers comprehensively.

I tried to keep things light by letting her know that Black people can now sit wherever they want on the bus. I explained that rules were changed after Rosa Parks refused to give up her seat and collaborated with other activists to protest the government to make things fairer for everyone. I also went on to assuage Briella's fears that there was anything wrong with being Black.

I reminded her that our entire family was Black—irrespective of hue—and assured her that no color was better than the other. I let her know that we can sit anywhere we want on planes, trains, buses, and any seats in our family-owned vehicles.

I don't know how the story of Rosa Parks and the Montgomery Bus Boycott was taught in Briella's first-grade class. However, I expect that her teachers used the best and most appropriate approach since she is enrolled in a private Christian school at the predominantly Black American church our family has attended since 2006.

However, given her conversation with Arielle, I'm sure she walked away from that lesson associating "Blackness" with disadvantage.

She intuitively didn't want to identify with being disadvantaged.

As a fiercely competitive and capable little girl, Briella is acutely aware of her intellect. She often declares herself a genius while voraciously consuming her Kumon math and reading worksheets. Daily. She is conditioned to want to win and have the "advantage." And earn praise from others for doing things well.

Bolanle also used the Kumon math and reading program worksheets growing up. Her Aunt, Adoline—one of the primary reasons she got exposed to Kumon as a child—owns a Kumon learning center. We obtained a waiver to enroll Briella in the Kumon learning program when she was 26-months old.

When we took Briella for her placement assessment, Aunt Adoline assumed we were overinflating her capabilities but was pleasantly surprised to see Briella sail through the initial evaluation.

Fortunately, we've been able to stick with the program since she started in 2017.

Briella continues to amaze us, Aunt Adoline and her teachers, with her capabilities.

When Arielle was 26-months old, we took her to the same Kumon learning center to complete her initial assessment. When we checked in, we were delighted to learn that because of Briella's performance in the Kumon math and reading program, the center had formally lowered the age of admission from 36-months to 24-months.

Our desire to heighten our children's awareness of Black excellence led us to buy a third of an acre and build a house in a gated estate community in Prince George's county.

Prince Georges County has the distinction of being the second wealthiest, majority Black county in America.

Although Prince George's county's Black residents represent some of the wealthiest Black households in America, the county still suffers from poor access to health care and poor health outcomes.

In 2020, Prince George's county had the highest number of COVID-19 infections in the State of Maryland.

Prince George's County has more than one hundred thousand fewer residents than neighboring, primarily White, and wealthier Montgomery County.

Prince George's county also experienced the highest COVID-19 death rate per capita. Prince George's county residents' poorer health outcomes pre-date COVID-19.

The county has historically led the state in the incidence of chronic illness and maternal mortality rates.

According to the 2019 Prince George's County Health Department Maternal and Infant Health Report, significant disparities persist between Black and non-Black maternal and infant mortality rates in Prince George's county.

In 2017, the same year Arielle was born, the infant mortality rate among Black infants born in Prince George's county was more than double the rate among Hispanic infants. From 2008 to 2017, pregnancy-related maternal mortality rates in Prince George's county were higher than the state average.

Black moms died at the highest rate in the state.

Those sobering statistics caused us to look elsewhere when we evaluated which hospitals we wanted to deliver our children. We decided to use hospitals in neighboring, mostly White, Howard, and Anne Arundel counties. Despite our best efforts, we still had to contend with condescending attitudes, premature dismissals of some concerns we raised, and shoddy work during our second delivery.

Shoddy work that we discovered while Bolanle was delivering our third child, Michelle.

Shoddy work that could have easily cost Bolanle her life.

A tragedy we avoided thanks to the brilliant work of the lead physician—a woman of color—that delivered Michelle. The lead physician dedicated the time necessary to repair the shoddy work from when Arielle was born.

She didn't rush off to the next thing.

Over the years, a gradual rise in Cesarean Section (C-Section) births has been recorded. According to the Centers for Disease Control and Prevention (CDC), more than 30-percent of all deliveries in America were completed via C-Section.

In 2019, states like Mississippi (38.5%), Louisiana (36.7%), and Florida (36.5%) all reported C-Section rates above 35-percent. The states with the lowest rates were Alaska (21.6%), Utah (23.1%), and Idaho (24%). The racial demographics of a particular state is one of the underlying factors responsible for the disparities in C-Section rates across America.

High C-Section rate states like Mississippi, Louisiana, and Florida have large populations of people of color.

Low C-Section rate states like Alaska, Utah, and Idaho have small populations of people of color.

One key factor associated with rising maternal morbidity is the increased use of C-Sections. In addition, women with low-risk pregnancies undergoing C-Sections are wasteful spending that has not led to better outcomes for infants or women.

According to the Centers for Medicare and Medicaid Services (CMS), Medicaid was the payment source for 42-percent of all 2018 births in America. Poverty is another factor associated with rising maternal morbidity.

Rising alongside C-Section rates has been the rate of pregnancy-related deaths.

CDC's Pregnancy Mortality Surveillance System (PMSS) reports that the rates of pregnancy-related deaths went from 7 out of 100,000 live births in 1987 to a ratio of 18 out of 100,000 live births in 2014.

Of the pregnancy-related deaths reported between 2014 and 2017, about <u>40-percent of the women who died from pregnancy-related complications were Black moms</u>.

Undergoing C-Sections have all the risks associated with any type of abdominal surgery. However, with C-Sections, those risks and complications can impact both the mom and the baby.

I posit that Black moms who are inappropriately recommended for C-Sections and have to contend with unpleasant environmental factors and racial trauma are predisposed to achieving worse outcomes when compared to White moms who don't have to deal with the same challenges.

Once a mom undergoes a C-Section, a C-Section is typically the only way she proceeds with future births. Moms that attempt a vaginal delivery after a C-Section have to contend with the risk of ruptures and hemorrhaging. Birthing teams prefer not to deal with those risks.

According to the PMSS, some of the leading causes of pregnancy-related deaths are Infection or sepsis, cardiomyopathy, and bleeding. They are leading causes associated chiefly with or exacerbated by C-Sections.

While there are many reasons for the rise in C-Section rates, one of the most despicable reasons is that C-Sections generate more revenue for provider organizations. C-Sections are also the more efficient approach for the delivering physician.

Although we didn't feel safe delivering any of our children in Prince George's county, we are glad to call the county home. We appreciate the demographic profile of the county we are proud to call home.

We remain hopeful that equitable, higher-value, consumer-centric care will become the future standard of care in Prince George's county. A higher-value standard of care that is actualized while retaining its Black majority.

I consider the gated estate community where we live <u>our safe space</u>.

As a Black man in America, the gated estate community where I live is like a sanctuary. I can take walks or go for a run at any time of the day or night without being fearful of racial profiling, being hunted by vigilantes, and gunned down like Ahmaud Arbery.

My heart breaks for Ahmaud and his family.

I hope his murderers are held accountable and punished accordingly.

It breaks my heart that only a tiny fraction of Black people in America are experiencing this safe space. It warms my heart when we take walks as a family and encounter diverse but mostly Black families also out for walks or bike rides within the gated estate community.

Although we are privileged to have our safe space, whenever I venture out of the gated estate community, I feel a slight tinge of fear. A feeling I've been trying to shake in the 5-years since construction on our home was completed and we moved in.

I hope one day the perimeter of where I consider a safe space in America expands for other Black people and me. Safe spaces where we can be our authentic selves without concerns of unnecessary exposure to Race-Based Traumatic Stress (RBTS).

Two Worlds Collide

"To be a Negro in this country and to be relatively conscious is to be in a rage almost all the time." – James Baldwin

Almost all the benefits of privilege I'd grown up with vanished when I immigrated to America in 2002.

In Nigeria, I lived in a mansion. In a gated community. I had my own room, with a closet.

We had a driver.

We had a gateman.

We had people that cleaned the house.

We had people that washed and ironed our clothes.

We had people that picked up our groceries and cooked our meals.

We had a lot of privileges.

After the ruling dictator—General Sani Abacha—threatened to arrest professors at the University of Ibadan in 1998, my parents moved our family from the University of Ibadan to a property they built. The mansion was built in a gated community, in an established housing estate.

When we arrived in America, my younger brother, Mayowa, and I shared a small room.

The room had an equally small closet.

Our apartment was in New Carrollton, Maryland.

I shared the three-bedroom apartment with my mother and three of my siblings.

The apartment was in a lower-income neighborhood in Prince George's County.

It was situated across the street from a shopping mall complex.

A Shoppers grocery store was the anchor tenant.

I was sad and angry.

I was ashamed because I had lost most of the privileges I grew up with.

I was determined to reacquire those privileges as quickly as possible.

As I transitioned to life in America, I went from encountering daily reminders of the privileges I enjoyed, to discovering all the different ways I was disadvantaged in America. For example, growing up, our driver dropped my siblings and me off at school by driving down Akinyele Road. A road named after King Akinyele, my father's uncle. That road was the main driveway into the International School of Ibadan (ISI).

ISI is the elite secondary school I attended for 6-years.

ISI is within the gated campus of the University of Ibadan.

Also infuriating was the disparity between the privileges our family name bestowed on me in Nigeria to the infamy I initially associated with the same name in America. I was clued into the infamy after introducing myself with my first and last name to a slightly older Black man at church. He chuckled. He asked if Akinyele was really my last name.

I told him it was and inquired why he asked.

I conducted an internet search of the name Akinyele.

I discovered that in America, our family name was primarily associated with a foul-mouthed rapper known for his grimy, explicit lyrics. I realized how much my "status" had diminished. I eventually realized that because I was Black, I wouldn't be able to replicate all the privileges I'd gotten accustomed to in Nigeria.

I believed I wouldn't be able to maximize my potential in America.

I was sad and angry.

I was determined to push the bounds of what was possible in America.

I was further dismayed while going through freshman registration at the Howard University student clinic. The college student calling out the names completely butchered the pronunciation of both my first and last names, causing the entire room to burst into laughter.

As folks in the room were roaring in laughter, I thought to myself, *"It must suck to be whoever that is."* At that moment, I also remembered a story my father told us growing up about linguistics tests used by Yoruba people to identify and detain or kill non-Yoruba's they encountered in Yoruba territory during the Nigerian Civil War—The Biafra war.

Unbeknownst to me, it was my name that they were announcing when the room burst into laughter.

When no one claimed the appointment spot, they crossed the name off the list and called the next name on the list. After an hour or so went by, I walked up to the registration desk to inquire how much longer I had to wait before my name was called. When I glanced at the clipboard, I discovered that my name had been crossed out already.

At that moment, I realized it was my name they called when the room erupted in laughter. I wrote down my name again.

This time, I wrote down Michael instead of Olaoluwa.

I channeled my inner Dorothy and muttered to myself, *"We ain't in Kansas no more, Toto."*

How any society treats names and accents is connected to social and tribal hierarchies like race and ethnicity. Dehumanizing treatment starts with small acts like openly mocking or ridiculing someone.

To avoid any additional challenges associated with my "accent" or America's linguistic shortcomings, I eventually decided to evolve my code-switching abilities.

I developed a generic American accent. It was helpful for time spent in academic and professional settings.

I developed an Ebonics accent. It was helpful for time spent interacting with folks in the pre-gentrified Shaw-Howard neighborhood in North-West Washington, D.C. The area where Howard University's campus is located.

Making matters worse, my father decided to remain in Nigeria.

He eventually let us know that he didn't want to restart his career or live full-time in America. His decision not to relocate came as a shock to us since his older brother, Professor Olusola Akinyele, decided in 1994 to relocate his family from Ibadan to Baltimore, Maryland.

I was angry at my father because I felt like his decision robbed me of the primary "top-cover" I relied on growing up. Top cover manifested in a well-connected father who could resolve any issue that came up. He was a well-connected father who enabled me to overcome almost any adversity I faced.

I was also confused by his decision because he lived in America in the 1970s while earning his Ph.D. at the University of Illinois at Urbana-Champaign. Later in the 1980s, he lived in Des Moines, Iowa. In Iowa, he collaborated on a research effort while on sabbatical from his primary job as a professor at the University of Ibadan.

While I don't know all that went into the calculus of his eventual decision to reside in Nigeria primarily, I assume he preferred continuing to enjoy his privileged status in Nigeria. And he didn't want to re-engage American White supremacy on a full-time basis.

Realizing I no longer had the "top cover" or "privilege" I had grown accustomed to, I chose to chart a new path.

I decided to focus on earning my way into positions of privilege in America. The fabled land of opportunity. I was single-minded back then. I wanted to accumulate sufficient wealth to replicate the life I'd grown accustomed to in Nigeria.

My parents instilled in us the mindset that devotion to our Christian faith and education would be the foundation for our success. They often reminded us that they didn't inherit any physical assets from their parents. They let us know that the investment made in their education, hard work, and strong networks was responsible for the economic success and status our family enjoyed. With that in mind, I focused on getting the best possible grades while earning money working full-time.

I didn't have to confront disadvantages unique to my "Blackness" until I started recruiting for full-time jobs during the fall semester of my senior year at Howard University.

My first traumatic exposure to "elitist White supremacy™" manifested with a "curveball question" from three White interviewers evaluating entry-level recruits for an economics consulting firm conducting first-round interviews on campus.

There I sat, barely three years removed from my privileged existence in Ibadan.

Trying to anticipate the next technical question I was going to be asked.

To my surprise and dismay, the next question was, "So, how do you feel about working with White people?"

Visibly taken aback by the nature of the question, it took what seemed like an eternity for me to compose myself and give the most politically correct answer I could muster.

We wrapped up the interview a couple of minutes later.

I had barely closed the door behind me before I heard all three interviewers burst into roaring laughter.

I felt humiliated.

I hoped no one else around me could hear them laughing.

I wondered how this could happen to me at Howard University.

I've since observed similar scenarios play out in popular culture. For example, in Black Math—episode eighteen, season four of the sitcom Black-ish—Dre (Anthony Anderson) had a flashback to when he was interviewing for a job after graduating from Howard University. Junior (Marcus Scribner) was deciding whether he should attend Howard University or Stanford University. Bow (Tracee Ellis Ross) reminded Dre of challenges he experienced looking for work with his Howard University degree.

The "curveball question" Dre received from his White interviewer was "Howard University, huh? What do they teach there, Black math?"

While Dre and his White interviewer both burst out laughing in response to the question, the thought bubble that appeared on the screen was Dre was reaching over the table while attempting to strangle the interviewer.

I wish the show and that episode existed back in 2005 when I was going through the interviewing process during my senior year. While I would have still been taken aback by the nature of the question, hopefully, I wouldn't have exhibited visible signs of extreme discomfort and unease. Exacerbating my discomfort was the calculus of trying to figure out the best way to respond to the question while being evaluated by a prospective employer.

The shame I felt at that moment still bothers me today.

I remain irritated that I let them get away with messing with me.

They got a good laugh out of it.

I imagine they likely shared with their colleagues the story of how they made a Black student squirm during a job interview.

Hoping to avoid replicating the trauma from that experience, I recalibrated my evaluation criteria for potential employers.

I made psychological safety the number one selection criteria. Employer brand value and compensation rounded out the top three selections. At the time, I was executing a 5-year plan to accomplish some early wins in my career. Early wins that would enable me to pursue an MBA at an elite business school.

I surmised that pre-MBA employer brand value and compensation wouldn't matter as much in the long run if miscreants at my pre-MBA employer derailed my career or undermined my self-confidence.

From that point forward, my revised standard became an unstated requirement to interact with Black people during the interview process. My nirvana saw Black people not just confined to supporting or junior roles at the potential employer's organization.

Most companies I interviewed with didn't meet that standard. Thankfully, the job market was booming in 2006. Fortunately, I received multiple job offers since I graduated magna cum laude with the highest cumulative Grade Point Average (GPA) in my major, economics.

I accepted an offer from Huron Consulting Group (Huron). I believed I would enjoy the work and also have a fair shot at climbing the corporate ladder at a brisk pace. I figured that since there was at least one Black person performing duties at every level of the company's Washington D.C. office, there weren't any glass ceilings for me to spend extra years chipping away at to advance.

There was Juliet, an Analyst and a fellow Howard alum.

Then Mahmoud, a Manager and fellow African immigrant.

And Tamika, a Managing Director in her thirties.

I first met Tamika during my final round interview in her well-appointed office. During the interview, I remember admiring her achievements and envisioning how I could lead a similar life in America later in my career.

I was also comforted knowing that Marc, the Jewish man who was the head of Huron's D.C. office at the time, was one of the people who sponsored Tamika's career before they decided to leave KPMG and join Huron to establish its D.C. office.

During my final round interview with Marc in his corner office, I took a mental note of his monogrammed cuffs and pocket square. I envisioned a future where I would don similar attire while engaging clients, helping to solve their problems.

I experienced a similar but publicly humiliating and more traumatizing episode during the Executive Challenge at Stanford University Graduate School of Business (GSB) in 2010.

The primarily White judging panel—all but the lone faculty member of South Asian descent—gave me feedback that I can only summarize as my "Blackness" made it impossible for them to trust me.

The faculty member was poised to give his feedback last.

He could see that I was flooded with emotions, visibly.

He chose not to provide any feedback.

The White judges exclusively gave me feedback on things I did that made them "uneasy."

Their comments ranged from "the combination of your bald head and broad shoulders."

To "your hand movements."

Then "high energy." Etcetera.

The hardest-hitting comment was, "your pitch made us uneasy. It felt very much like a used car salesman trying to sell us a lemon."

There I was, dressed in my black pinstripe three-piece suit sans pocket square, trying to channel my inner Gordon Gekko. Earlier that day, my Black MBA student mentor advised me to remove my pocket square.

These White judges reacted to me like I was trying to sell them fake Rolexes outside of a bodega in Queens, New York. The entire scene played out in front of my primarily White study group and the White second-year MBA student coaching us.

None of the feedback was about the product or idea. The White judges couldn't see past my "Blackness."

The countless times I have relived the humiliation I felt in that moment and the trauma of that experience, I still wonder why the people representing Stanford didn't help me. I wonder why the faculty member on the judging panel or the second-year MBA student who saw me visibly getting crushed by the feedback didn't pull me aside and refer me to whatever counseling service was available. I even attempted to bring it up doing our debrief huddle before the next round of pitching. Awkward silence. Crickets.

Part of me initially assumed I was part of some "Stanford Experiment."

I expected enlightenment at the end of the GSB Executive Challenge.

No revelatory enlightenment happened.

The trauma of my GSB Executive Challenge experience worsened as I witnessed non-Black classmates get positive feedback for their "high-energy" pitches and "powerfully descriptive hand movements."

The only feedback—mostly positive—I received related to the product idea I was pitching came from the Black alumni observer who evaluated my pitch from the side of the room.

She wasn't "intimidated" by my energy. My physical features. My hand movements.

Representation matters.

My confidence evaporated after the GSB Executive Challenge.

Imposter syndrome kicked into high gear.

I slowly slipped into a depressed state.

I spent most of my time alone in my room in the Munger residential building.

I largely avoided social interactions

I assumed word got out about the feedback I received.

I assumed no one would want to collaborate with a guy that could elicit such a response from investors and senior executives in the heart of Silicon Valley.

I felt so alone, being so far away from home and my support system. Bolanle. My family in Maryland. Mentors. My church family.

Unsupported.

Sad and angry.

Humiliated.

Alone.

I was devastated in the weeks that followed my GSB Executive Challenge experience.

To make matters worse, I couldn't shake the sinking feeling that I couldn't gain equal access to the same opportunities as my mostly White classmates no matter what I did. The optimism with which I viewed what was possible because I earned my MBA from the top-ranked business school in the world, and the resulting network effect...shattered.

As the months turned into quarters, I helplessly watched the rest of my first year at the GSB spiral.

Thankfully, during my second year, I talked through some of the trauma and issues I carried with me while engaging classmates in the T-Group—Touchy-Feely—I was assigned in my Interpersonal Dynamics class.

I was often prepared to endure primal White supremacy™, typically manifested when I frequently got pulled over driving my BMW sedan. I currently drive a Honda minivan and haven't gotten pulled over yet. Fingers crossed.

It took me a while to fully comprehend the construct of elitist White supremacy™.

Elite organizations and institutions with an overrepresentation of White males in positions of authority or influence are the quintessential harbingers of elitist White supremacy™.

An irritating reminder of the pervasiveness of this malaise is that in 2021, most senior Executive Officers—top-5 most powerful Executives—of Fortune 500 and FTSE 100 companies have almost no Black people and only a few women in their ranks.

Other institutions labeled "Liberal" like academic Institutions of higher learning continue to primarily advance White males to tenured faculty positions and different influential positions in their ecosystem.

I assume the manifestation of this malaise is why the Boston area, with its cluster of elite academic institutions, is considered the "South" of the North East.

The controversy surrounding Professor Cornel West not being offered a tenured faculty position at Harvard University serves as a reminder of the continued existence of this problem.

Harvard didn't award Professor West tenure.

He eventually left.

Since some American media platforms are enablers of the same elitist White supremacy™, they are reluctant to shine a persistent, meaningful light on this problem or promote viable paths to change.

Additional manifestations of elitist White supremacy™ persisted throughout the rest of my professional career. Another experience stemmed from the inadvertent disclosure of my royal heritage during my pre-MBA consulting days.

While huddled in a team room with coworkers completing a forensic review of emails and financials from a litigation case we were working on, a coworker came across one of the infamous "Nigerian Prince" emails.

After he reviewed the email, he wondered out loud how folks fell for these scams since each email was from a different "Prince."

I explained how it was easy to have so many different "Nigerian Princes." Nigeria is a collection of hundreds of tribes and kingdoms amalgamated to benefit the British Empire and not its indigenous people.

While the design benefited the British Empire, it undermined Nigeria's progress and its eventual system of government.

I'd barely gotten done with my explanation before one of my coworkers said, "so you're a Nigerian Prince? Guess we have to start screening your emails more carefully."

The room erupted in laughter in response to his statement.

Though mildly irritated, I took it in stride because I was friendly with all of my coworkers in the room, and I didn't perceive his comment as being laced with malice or designed to humiliate me.

I still find it unbelievable that Nigeria—the most populous Black nation globally—has been branded as a nation of fraudsters and financial crime masterminds by the American media industrial complex.

It's more likely that the incidence of financial crime in Nigeria and by Nigerians is proportional to rates seen in other nations.

One out of every six Africans is Nigerian. There's a high probability that if an African is in the mix, the African is of Nigerian descent.

Most of the advance-fee fraud emails originated from other countries, including countries in Eastern Europe. But like everything else filtered through the lens of White supremacy, the propaganda machine stands ready to magnify Black association with criminality and consequently minimize White association with crime.

From a financial impact standpoint, the fraud perpetrated by Bernie Madoff or the criminals that orchestrated the Enron scandal inflicted more economic destruction on more Americans than the combination of all the Nigerians involved in advance-fee fraud schemes ever did.

Given that reality, it would be a bit more logical for American society to be more fearful and seek to raise awareness of Ponzi schemes and corporate fraud. Not advance-fee fraud.

I suppose that situation is similar to the reality that police have murdered more Black people accused of petty theft or using counterfeit currency than the number of primarily White "dudes" who orchestrated the 2008 financial crisis.

The 2008 financial crisis was an avoidable calamity that robbed millions of ordinary Americans of their net worth and future economic well-being. Economic malaise caused by thieving White "dudes."

Thieving White "dudes" that never saw the end of a cop's gun.

Thieving White "dudes" that never saw the inside of a jail cell.

Thieving White "dudes" that never saw the inside of a courtroom.

Thieving White "dudes" that are still thieving. Lobbying. Unencumbered. Lethal.

Elitist White supremacists typically choose to demonstrate their "allyship" to the cause of addressing racial injustice by denouncing manifestations of primal White supremacy™.

They perform their "allyship" while appearing willfully ignorant of the elitist White supremacy™ they promote in their own lives. Daily.

For example, elitist White supremacists that are "ultra-woke" members of the Liberal Left are quick to denounce primal White supremacists as "deplorable." They eagerly condemn and highlight recorded racial injustices that primal White supremacists inflict on people of color. Racial injustices focused on needs at the base of Maslow's pyramid.

However, the manifestations of White supremacy that elitist White supremacists traumatize people of color with are focused on needs at the top of Maslow's pyramid.

They deter people of color from meeting their psychological needs.

They deter them from achieving self-actualization in their desired professional pursuits.

They deter them from maximizing their potential.

Since being sound in mind and body is required to achieve optimal health outcomes, I believe that injustice is injustice. White supremacy is White supremacy.

The primal side <u>traumatizes the body</u>.

The elitist side <u>traumatizes the mind</u>.

Primal White supremacy™ and elitist White supremacy™ are two sides of the same coin.

When elitist White supremacists condemn primal White supremacists, calls for racial justice reforms ring hollow. Those calls for racial justice typically have a limited impact.

If elitist White supremacists genuinely care about advancing racial justice reforms, they should first look within the organizations and institutions they control.

They should focus on dismantling the systemic racism within.

Only then would a modicum of "moral high ground" manifest. And the opportunity to demonstrate to primal White supremacists that elitist White supremacists are willing to reform the institutions that primarily benefit elitist White supremacists.

For example, although the US civil war was about slavery, ending racial discrimination and dismantling structural racism wasn't the Union army's goal. Instead, the focus of the Union army was on controlling the South by weakening, delegitimizing, and dismantling their source of economic wealth and power—unpaid labor of enslaved people from Africa.

Similarly, gun ownership—privileges of "open carry," "stand your ground," etcetera—and the law enforcement industrial complex are institutions that primal White supremacists use to oppress and traumatize Black people.

Chastisement from elitist White supremacists on the racial injustices propagated by primal White supremacists rings hollow. It rings hollow because those same elitist White supremacists aren't making meaningful progress on efforts to reform organizations and institutions they control.

Organizations and institutions that primarily benefit elitist White supremacists.

The Bible says in Matthew Chapter 7 verse 5, "you hypocrite! First, take the beam out of your eye, and then you will see clearly to remove the speck from your brother's eye."

Resonant of a quote from Malcolm X, "The White Liberal differs from the White Conservative only in one way: the Liberal is more deceitful than the Conservative. Both want power, but the White liberal is the one who has perfected the art of posing as the Negro's friend and benefactor."

I acknowledge that the trauma inflicted by primal White supremacists on Black people can often lead to physical death. However, the White supremacists uniquely positioned to empower Black people to close the wealth gap and gain socioeconomic might are the elitist ones.

Black people must gain socioeconomic might that is sufficient to reform the legislature.

We must reform legislatures willing to cover up atrocities committed by state-sanctioned institutions.

Those state-sanctioned institutions traumatize Black people.

They inequitably incarcerate Black people.

They cause the physical death of Black people.

"I have almost reached the regrettable conclusion that the Negro's greatest stumbling block in his stride toward freedom is not the Ku Klux Klanner, but the White moderate, who is more devoted to 'order' than to justice."
– Rev. Dr. Martin Luther King Jr.

Summary of My Career Journey

"The greatest waste...is failure to use the abilities of people... to learn about their frustrations and about the contributions that they are eager to make." – W. Edwards Deming

I started my career managing physician practices in the Washington, D.C. metro area while I was in my sophomore year studying economics at Howard University. I transitioned to a role in management consulting after graduation. I spent several years working on, and leading teams focused on developing and implementing solutions to strategic and operational challenges facing organizations of all sizes.

I've advised health systems, physician groups, academic medical centers, health plans, pharmaceutical companies, pharmacy benefit managers, and a Medicaid agency in the American health care industry. I often grew frustrated and felt dissatisfied with some of the challenges that came with the work-life of a management consultant. I took it in stride because I was learning from each experience, rapidly progressing through my career, and earning competitive compensation. I also earned non-financial rewards from all the travel associated with the job.

My outlook changed on February 27, 2014, after receiving a call from my brother, Josiah. Clearly shaken and quietly sobbing, he told me our father had passed away from a medical incident while on work-related travel at a conference in Abuja, Nigeria.

I still don't remember what else we said during our call, but I remember being in shock, telling him to take care, and quietly returning to the conference room where I worked on a slide deck for a meeting later that day. I was away from home at a client site in North Carolina when I received the call from my brother. I didn't know how to process the information I just received but was glad it was a Thursday. The typical fly-back day for management consultants is Thursday, and I was flying home to Maryland later that day.

My father passed away at 67. He was an accomplished professional with a distinguished and productive career spanning academia, non-governmental organizations, and international economic development organizations. While I continue to strive to develop a similarly impactful and globally relevant career, I hope to eclipse the number of years he spent alive because I would like to spend more time enjoying the fruits of my labor. I would also like to enjoy some quality time in whole or semi-retirement before transitioning to the afterlife. It still saddens me when I internalize the reality that my children will never meet my father. Despite our pleas for him to retire and relax after his 65th birthday, he indicated he would do so at 70, a birthday milestone he never actualized.

I eventually pieced together the details surrounding my father's passing in the weeks following the call with my brother, Josiah. My father suffered a pulmonary embolism, and the care team that tried to help him did not know his medical or recent travel history. The care team also didn't contact his primary care physician or family members. I can only assume the care team that attended to him at the hospital focused on making his transition from life to death as painless as possible.

I will always wonder if the outcome of his final health care encounter would have been any different if his care team had access to his medical and recent travel history. Or if his primary care physician and family members were alerted when he initially showed signs of distress. I also wonder if the outcome would have been different if he was empowered with tools and resources to provide better self-care. I'd like to imagine that proper self-care would've prevented or helped identify early the blood clot that made its way to his lungs and caused the pulmonary embolism that ultimately took his life.

After his funeral, I was burdened with grief and a burning desire to honor his legacy with my career. I made up my mind to use my health care knowledge to create a global health care ecosystem where care teams or individuals would have convenient and affordable access to helpful information, tools, and resources. Valuable assets that help them achieve the best possible health outcomes. Those health outcomes are guided by leading evidence-based guidelines for diagnosis and treatment.

After eighteen months of reflecting and exploring different avenues to pursue my goal of building an impactful and mission-focused career, in March 2016, I accepted a role at the Laura and John Arnold Foundation as the Director of Venture Development – Health Care. I was very excited when I signed my offer letter even though accepting the job meant taking a six-figure pay cut to my total compensation as a management consultant. Nevertheless, I was excited because at that moment, I envisioned a career working for a billionaire couple focused on curing societal problems and fixing market failures. I initially viewed the opportunity as a "dream come true" and a "forever job" I could settle into as I pursued a career of meaning and impact.

Unfortunately, the honeymoon phase quickly faded. I eventually realized the limitations of effecting meaningful change from a platform of philanthropy. My "aha" moment came at an invitation-only gathering of healthcare-focused foundations in New York City later that summer.

Representatives of several foundations with combined assets of more than 10 billion dollars and annual disbursements of approximately 500 million dollars converged in a conference room at the host foundation's office. Our conversation quickly shifted from whatever narrow health reform problem we were supposed to be discussing to everyone chiming in about their hopes and dreams for a new version of an American health care ecosystem that would deliver more value for consumers and taxpayers. The reality implicitly and explicitly acknowledged in the room was that efforts the different foundations had funded in the past, currently had underway or planned for the immediate future, had no chance of catalyzing the creation of the American health care ecosystem we all envisioned.

Further, as one of the youngest people in the room and the only Black person, it was hard for me to imagine building a fulfilling career by staying on this path in the long run. I could see the defeated looks on the faces of equally passionate and more seasoned folks in the room. They had spent several years, for some, decades of their life, working to reform the American health care ecosystem with little impact realized.

Exacerbating my frustrations were work-life balance challenges associated with some unanticipated organizational dynamics I had to contend with while working at the foundation. My time at the foundation came to an end eight months after I started. Though my time working full-time in philanthropy was short-lived, I learned a great deal from the exposure. I made life-long friends and business acquaintances through the experience.

My appointment to the Lymphoma Research Foundation (LRF) Board of Directors occurred in November 2016. I am honored to still serve, supporting the mission of funding research to find a cure and helping those touched by the disease. While I currently cannot find fulfillment in a full-time career in philanthropy, I appreciate the continued opportunities to effect change through philanthropy. I continue learning about practical approaches consumer advocacy organizations utilize to serve their constituents and fulfill their mission.

I also started independent advisory work through The Maximizer Group, a limited liability company I formed in 2007 to explore investment opportunities and entrepreneurial pursuits.

I was hired into the U.S. Department of Veterans Affairs (VA) in August 2017 as a Senior Advisor to the Deputy Undersecretary for Health for Operations and Management (DUSHOM). The DUSHOM was the career official stationed in VA Central Office that all Veteran Integrated Service Network (VISN) Directors reported. Given its massive budget, policy, and regulatory influence, the nationwide scope of operations, and the noble mission of serving our nation's heroes, I initially viewed the VA as the ideal platform to effect meaningful change across the American health care ecosystem. The VA is a closed system capable of executing its mission without contending with all the broader American health care ecosystem constraints.

I eventually realized that with changes to agency leadership every four years—even in times of transition that kept the same political party in power—, there was a resetting of priorities and often a change in direction.

Partisan modifications to established pathways often traumatize career civil servants. According to long-tenured senior VA staff, the time I spent at the VA was particularly tumultuous, with significantly greater direction and leadership changes than typical.

The harsh reality of the limitations of working inside government dawned on me during a conversation with a long-tenured senior executive at the VA who told me the first year and last year of every administration is basically "dead-time" for new initiatives. I found this reality very hard to accept. Primarily because establishing the VA Innovation Center (VIC) to create and scale new initiatives was my job. New Administrations are typically focused on installing new leadership at the agencies during the first year and focused on upcoming elections or transitioning out of government during the last year.

After my third daughter, Michelle, was born in February 2020, I spent time pondering whether I should settle into a career as a civil servant. I had recently earned an appointment to the Senior Executive Service (SES) ranks in 2019. I ultimately attained a level-3 SES position after leading the VIC in an acting capacity for almost two years. The level-3 SES position in the civil service is equivalent to the Lieutenant General rank in the military. According to the Office of Personnel Management (OPM), SES is a corps of executives selected for their leadership qualifications, serving in key positions just below the top

Presidential appointees as a link between them and the rest of the federal (civil service) workforce.

At 36, I was the youngest Black Title-5 SES at the VA. This reality caused me to envision additional power and influence I could wield by ascending to increasingly senior roles at the VA in the ensuing years.

Unfortunately, the pandemic wore on, and the Black Lives Matter (BLM) protests hit a fever pitch. The murders of George Floyd and Breonna Taylor by police and the attempted murder of Christian Cooper—the Black bird watcher in Central Park—by a White "dudette" were the turning point for me. I spent a lot of time reflecting on how my children would regard my actions when we talked about the events of this period later in the future.

Also on my mind was the #EndSARS movement and protests occurring in Nigeria. Similar to the BLM movement, the #EndSARS movement centered on fighting against injustices suffered by mostly Black men at the hands of state-sanctioned forces. With the #EndSARS movement, it was the Nigerian Police Force.

My desire to be well-regarded and respected by my wife, Bolanle, and our children, challenge me to be a better person, husband, and father. My children, like most, are innately wired to dislike being mistreated or seeing people they care about suffer. As such, I knew that if I were to remain a hero and a man of character in their eyes, I would need to have a compelling narrative when we inevitably have future discussions as a family. When our children are much older. About the actions I took while the coronavirus pandemic was raging. And people around the globe were protesting racial injustice against Black people in America.

Like many, I have lost both people I care about and casual acquaintances to the coronavirus pandemic. In the spring of 2020, as the pandemic continued to spread across America, it lay bare the inequities and disparities in the American health care ecosystem. I often felt frustrated in my role leading the VA Innovation Center (VIC) since the established funding, governance process, and mission focus didn't allow for our work to be as responsive or impactful during the ongoing crisis. Exacerbating my frustration was the departure of the political appointee boss who hired me away from my role at the Veterans Health Administration (VHA). Melissa, the Assistant Secretary for Enterprise Integration (OEI), left the VA to return to a position in the private sector.

Her replacement, Karen, was concurrently serving as the Chief Acquisition Officer of the VA. It was clear from the onset that Karen would be overwhelmed trying to manage both offices. In the weeks following her appointment to lead OEI, it became abundantly clear that leaning forward on innovative initiatives that my office was established to pursue would never be top of mind for her to advocate for or advance, especially in an election year.

I also discovered that pursuing initiatives focused on exploring solutions to suicide prevention, the number one clinical priority of the VA, wasn't immune to the political and organizational dynamics that were prevalent at the time.

In the summer of 2020, President Trump orchestrated a now-infamous photo opportunity in front of the historic St. John's Church damaged in the aftermath of the Black Lives Matter (BLM) protests. My former office was in VA's Central Office (VACO) building next to the historic St. John's Church. The VACO building was also damaged. Soon after, the Trump Administration started pushing for a return to "normalcy" by directing senior leaders and some staff across the federal government to come and work in the office.

I vividly remember when the conversation occurred among the OEI leadership team, which Karen led at the time. As folks started raising concerns they had about coming into the office, Karen said, "I like my SES's in the office." When she said that, I remember thinking: *Lincoln abolished slavery, you don't own us. We serve the people.* Since all the other SES's on the call were being sheepish, I chimed in by reiterating the obvious. Our teams are virtual. Are you asking us to come into the office and telework from inside our respective offices?

I also indicated that my family had been taking every precaution and only leaving the house for emergencies or groceries. We had very stringent protocols in place since I have a preexisting condition. Hypertension. A wife completing her cardiology fellowship and three children under five. Two needed hands-on support with distance learning and the third was an infant. As an essential worker, Bolanle could help cover the COVID Cardiac Intensive Care Unit (ICU) at the health system where she worked. Further, with the alarming rates of women dropping out of the workforce during the ongoing pandemic, I wanted to prepare our household to primarily support the demands of Bolanle's career during the pandemic.

Across multiple generations of the Akinyele family, the women in the family have routinely sacrificed their career aspirations. I witnessed the challenges associated with that malaise growing up and committed to being the spouse to make career sacrifices to enable my wife to actualize her career aspirations.

Since graduating summa cum laude from Howard University in 2009 with the highest cumulative Grade Point Average (GPA) across all majors in the Division of Allied Health Sciences, Bolanle has been executing a 12-year plan to complete her medical and public health training. 2021 is the year she will complete her formal Professional Medical Training (PMT) process. Falling short or tripping with the finish line in sight wasn't an option we were willing to entertain.

In addition to being a wonderful wife, she is an amazing mother to our three beautiful daughters. Being married to me isn't a cakewalk. It isn't a net negative experience, but I'll be the first to admit that she puts up with a lot☺. Evolving a marriage to good requires hard work.

Bolanle was also completing the final year of her cardiology fellowship, studying to take her cardiology board exams later that fall, conducting clinical research, and concurrently completing her Master's in Public Health (MPH) coursework and a related global health research project. She remains the most exceptional person I know and the preeminent manifestation of beauty and brains embodied in one person.

Beyond concerns for our family's safety, any time either of us spent away from the house exacerbated the strain childcare and eldercare placed on our household. I also tried explaining to Karen that both my mother, Ayoni, who lived with us, and my mother-in-law, Barbara, who was visiting from Nigeria, were also household members. As usual, after Michelle was born, Barbara stepped away from the businesses she runs with my father-in-law, Abdul, in Nigeria to continue her tradition of caring for her grandchildren in the first few months of their lives.

Both Ayoni and Barbara, who helped care for Michelle, were over 65. According to the Centers for Disease Control and Prevention (CDC), they also had preexisting conditions that might put them at an increased risk for severe illness from the virus that causes COVID-19. An additional strain was on the horizon because Barbara returned to Nigeria the first week of September. And Briella was returning to school and entering an era of distance learning.

Finally, I also highlighted the risks of a Black man commuting to downtown D.C. and being near the White House at a time when protesters were spontaneously clashing. Anti-riot police were often overly aggressive, especially towards Black men. Being the lone Black male SES voice in most meetings (including this one), I always felt burdened to speak out on specific issues. In addition to the risks of exposure to COVID-19 or the probability of physical harm from exposure to anti-riot police or clashing protesters, secretly, I also didn't want to confront the shame of strolling past my fellow citizens protesting racial injustice. Strolling by, going about my business, walking into a federal building I didn't need to be in, one where social distancing and mask-wearing were optional.

My concerns fell on deaf ears as Karen retorted, "I don't know why they are protesting. If they want a change, they should go and vote." In my mind, I was thinking: *how does this White "dudette" from West Virginia not know about the suppression of the votes of people of color in America?*

In reality, I assume she understood that while the talking point is "they should go and vote," the dominant strategy employed by American institutions is to make it extremely hard for certain members of the American electorate to exercise their right to vote.

Karen shared that she had two sons-in-law who worked in law enforcement in Maryland. I realized she was indicating what side of the issue she was on. For a fleeting moment, I initially viewed her comment as a veiled threat. I quickly reminded myself that there was zero chance she would've bothered to remember that I lived in Maryland.

After reflecting on her comments, it became abundantly clear that she wasn't going to be empathetic to my concerns. Similarly, I had no desire to empathize with her point of view. Although our general attitude towards the other person's perspective was similar, I'm not equating the divergent viewpoints. I was advocating for my physical safety and reduced work-related strain on my household. Karen, a political appointee, was focused on "not getting in trouble" with the "10th Floor." The "10th Floor" is a reference to Secretary Wilkie's inner circle.

While I was enduring hostilities in my OEI leadership meetings and subsequent interactions with Karen, I was fortunate to be in a position to create a safe space for the diverse team that supported the innovation office I led. Our diverse innovation team talked about our varied experiences with racial injustice and shared our perspectives on the ongoing civil unrest. The team appreciated having the opportunity to discuss racial justice issues with their co-workers instead of awkwardly interacting like nothing out of the ordinary was happening in the real world.

When an employee, even an SES, resists their boss' direction, things don't typically take a turn for the better. I usually heed the words of Dave Burris, my mentor of 15-years and one of my three surrogate American dads, whenever I flirt with taking a stand, "you can only set yourself on fire once. After that, you're toast." My other two American dads are my pastor of 15-years and my brother-in-law, Ajibola Akinyemi, also a Howard University alum. I knew the hammer was coming after I stood my ground by refusing to telework from inside my office.

After Karen directed the SES's in OEI to telework from inside their office frequently, things started to unravel for my office. Initiatives the innovation office I led was working on were slow-rolled. Like the Suicide Prevention Grand Challenge, my requests to onboard new staff and obligate funding to support the Suicide Prevention Grand Challenge.

As the toxicity of my work environment worsened, microaggressions like Karen insisting on calling me "Mike," which she knows I dislike, resurfaced. I know she knew because I asked the OEI Chief of Staff to let her know. And she confirmed she relayed the message. I'm not a pet. I cherish the actual names my grandfather bestowed on me. Since I knew Karen wouldn't be bothered to learn how to pronounce my last name, I figured she could at least consistently use my actual first name. Michael.

During my time at the VA, I had read Government Accountability Office (GAO) reports. I heard rumors of employees getting railroaded or set up to "catch a case" with the VA Office of Inspector General (OIG). Further, in 2017, Congress passed, and President Trump enacted the VA Accountability and Whistleblower Protection Act. They named the law in honor of a former VA employee, Dr. Chris Kirkpatrick. He was a 38-year-old clinical psychologist who shot himself in the head after being fired from the Tomah VA Medical Center. Accounts surrounding his death indicate that he endured retaliation for challenging management about treatment provided at the center.

They eventually terminated Chris after putting him through the retaliatory ringer. He was devastated by the termination and also burdened with significant student debt. He took his life on the same day as his termination.

With Chris' experience in mind, I researched tactics used in the federal government to retaliate against "troublemakers." I scrutinized subsequent incidents or interactions I considered abnormal. I was at a heightened alert for any indication that the staff or contractors supporting the VIC were in cahoots against me. I eventually decided it wasn't worth it to pile on the stress of wondering if people I worked with "were out to get me."

In preparation for what increasingly seemed like my inevitable departure, I requested clearance from the VA Senior Ethics Official to advise startup companies during my personal time. I also started bringing up succession planning in discussions with my boss and other OEI senior leaders. I made it clear I was no longer interested in my job since I wasn't allowed to do it.

I contemplated "kissing the ring" and regressing to a compromised position. However, I was repulsed by the thought of "crawling on my knees" in an effort I expected would require me to present myself as a slightly dim-witted, always cheerful, non-assertive Black man. A caricature I figured a White "dudette" literally named Karen would be better accustomed to interacting with from her supervisory perch.

I decided against that approach and reasserted my initial decision to bring my authentic self to work. Walking with my head held high, I knew I was ok with whatever consequences may come. Of primary import was maintaining my integrity and my family's safety. Dying on the job or dying because of a job isn't part of my life goals.

All but one other OEI SES dialed into our leadership video calls from inside their office in the weeks that followed. My fellow holdout recently survived a heart attack and was counting down the time to retirement. Those who joined from inside their offices wore oversized American flag pins and professed their patriotism for some reason. I kid, I know the reason they were all doing this; they were fearful of losing favor with "the boss."

As they chimed in with their updates, I could see Karen beaming, clearly impressed with herself that she had the power to compel these folks to come and sit in their office during a pandemic when they had no justifiable reason to be in the building. As I sat in those meetings, I pondered what my future career could look like if I stayed in the civil service. I knew I had no desire to find myself in my mid-forties or beyond, kowtowing to the whims of every political appointee supervisor and Administration sycophant. People that would cycle through VA leadership every couple of years.

My tenure leading the VA Innovation Center ended in September 2020. My time came to a close after completing 3-years of the most challenging, mission-focused, and rewarding work I have ever led. I remain humbled and honored to have led the effort to establish the Center for Innovation for Care and Payment at the VA.

Inclusion of the Center in the VA MISSION Act of 2018 was critical. Lawmakers envisioned that the Center would stand as VA's version of the CMS Innovation Center created by the Affordable Care Act of 2010. I am proud of the infrastructure we built and the waiver request authorities we permanently retained for the Department. Properly wielded, VA's waiver request authority will enable the acceleration of regulation or policy-inspired innovation for years to come.

While my departure was bittersweet, I acknowledge that no one can "finish the work of innovation" at any organization but rather accomplish what we can, for as long as possible, then pass the baton. I remain confident that the thousands of change agents and innovators that continue to work at the VA will keep the fire burning for decades to come. Despite my departure from the VA, I remain committed to pursuing opportunities to serve our nation's heroes while continuing to support the VA's mission wherever and whenever I can.

As we headed into the fall flu season of 2020 with the COVID-19 pandemic still raging, I felt compelled to explore additional opportunities and approaches to achieving an outsized impact on the most significant number of lives.

As the months wore on, I often wondered if I would ever find a mission-oriented organization to pursue my self-appointed "calling" to create a global health care ecosystem designed to deliver value to consumers and taxpayers.

I've since settled on a path of entrepreneurship and a pivot back to my first love: capitalism. With my entrepreneurial pursuits, I seek to embody what I classify as a "benevolent capitalist^{TM}." A person who seeks to maximize personal gain and aggressively uses their accumulated wealth to make the world a better place.

To get started on this journey of benevolent capitalism, I've decided to invest my time and resources into several initiatives and new ventures designed to support my quest to invent the future of health care.

My primary focus is on exploring opportunities to raise a venture capital fund to invest in solutions that will power the future of health care delivery and payments.

I'm also pursuing opportunities to tap into the power of media to inspire action that I hope leads us to the "Promised Land:" a simple, affordable, and equitable American health care ecosystem that works for all Americans.

An American health care ecosystem that isn't designed to undermine American prosperity.

Perils of Elevating Mediocrity

"It is certain, in any case, that ignorance, allied with power, is the most ferocious enemy justice can have." – James Baldwin

Despite its history of genocide, slavery, racism, exploitation, bigotry, crazy politics, and trauma-inducing manifestations of White supremacy, I still believe that America is a great country. A nation with the potential to be the greatest country on earth of all time.

I hold this belief because, in America, the condition of one's birth doesn't always, and singularly, determine the outcome of one's life. But the possibility inherent in the American experiment is double-edged. America can inflict multi-generational harm on groups or individuals while also having the same power to bestow benefits, favor, and opportunity to the same groups or individuals. The outcome of this capacity rests upon American democracy when the electorate exercises their right to vote and elects new leaders to enact the people's will.

I wouldn't have achieved as much as I have in the 18-years I've lived in the United States if I immigrated to other developed nations instead. I wouldn't have made as much headway in the United Kingdom, Spain, Portugal, France, Italy, or any other country where elitist White supremacy™ continues to strengthen even as their respective economies and ivory towers crumble.

Though great, the United States is barely scratching the surface on maximizing its true potential, domestically or globally. The United States can step into exceptional greatness by redesigning American institutions to serve all Americans equitably.

If reform efforts remain beholden to special interests and enablers of White supremacy, I fear that America won't live up to its full potential. If the status quo is maintained or current trends persist, America will become increasingly hostile towards people of color and less relevant globally.

Manifestations of American White supremacy abound beyond its borders in an attempt to influence global affairs.

The American media industrial complex plays its part in promoting White supremacy across the globe by pushing the propaganda that "dark" is evil and "light" is good, helping to fan the flames of colorism and anti-Black sentiment worldwide. The use of the term "industrial complex" within the context of the U.S. military gained popularity after a warning on its damaging impact was highlighted in the farewell address of President Dwight D. Eisenhower on January 17, 1961.

Industrial complexes are particularly treacherous because they rest on relationships that include political contributions, political approval for spending, corporate lobbying, oversight of the industry, procurement, funding, and resource flows across private and government contractors, Congress, and the Executive branch.

The Judicial branch is getting roped into co-opting the growth and influence of industrial complexes across America. That unfortunate reality is highlighting how dire the current situation is.

The most insidious manifestation of this propaganda occurs when the word "black" is attached to harmful things that aren't even dark, supporting the notion that our global society should fear or mistrust all that is black or dark.

For example, why is "clear ice," which is treacherous to drive on, referred to by the media as "black ice"? Not all driving surfaces are covered with black asphalt, <u>the excuse</u>. So the use of the word "black" isn't universally applicable while using the word "clear" is.

The American media industrial complex also attempts to condition the masses to minimize harmful or criminal activity that has been "Whitewashed." Sanitized as being less harmful or unlawful. For example, "White lies," "White-collar crime."

There is some historical context for this propaganda, though. According to the Encyclopedia Britannica, the word "Whitewash" was first used in the late 1500s and is a metaphor meaning—to gloss over or cover up vices, crimes, or scandals or exonerate using a perfunctory investigation or biased presentation of data. In lay terms:

If a White person does it, it must be inherently right.

If a person of color does it, it must be inherently wrong.

While the effects of Whitewashing on world history, popular culture, and religion have been studied and publicized, I believe additional work is required to understand the negative impacts of Whitewashing. Primarily when protecting scandalous behavior or glossing over a reputation shrouded in controversy.

If extensively studied, I suspect we would find harmful effects in White people and people of color alike. Exposure to this type of propaganda is detrimental to everyone in the long run.

I posit that the harmful effects of the propaganda result in conditioned thinking that typically manifests as White people who feel like they can do no wrong because they don't experience full or any consequences for their harmful actions. In people of color, I assume the conditioned thinking typically manifests as suppressed ambition or self-loathing that can result in an identity crisis, mental stress, and loss of motivation.

Suppose skin color is considered essential to identifying as pious or criminal. In that case, White people who feel "imbued" with the color of "righteousness" may feel like whatever they do is right, while Black people who feel "imbued" with the color of "evil" may feel like they are unqualified or unable to achieve "righteousness."

In my experience, it takes a significant amount of self-awareness, self-love, and critical thinking to overcome the conditioned thinking propagated by Whitewashing.

The most toxic manifestation of the promotion of White supremacy by the American media industrial complex remains the on-screen fantasy that the "heroes," "leaders," and "problem-solvers" amongst us are almost always White males. Such narratives have translated into far-fetched plotlines like the Last Samurai, The Great Wall, and other such nonsense. Tom Cruise and Matt Damon, guys, you don't have to say yes to every script.

Via its pervasive content and distribution channels, American media propaganda promotes the notion that because of their "White maleness," mediocre White "dudes" are entitled to positions of power and authority. Such propaganda's toxic result reinforces the "delusions of grandeur" and sentiments of unearned "exceptionalism" that many White males have.

A separate but related cancer exacerbating this calamity is the modern American culture of racking up "participation trophies" and filling children's heads with the malarkey that every American is exceptional.

These delusional mindsets are challenged by the realities of an American economy falling behind in the global transition to the next industrial revolution.

When the "rubber meets the road," White "dudes" whose mediocre performance often gets celebrated as exceptional across generations eventually realize their life can't measure up to the fantasy of ubiquitous White exceptionalism.

Manifestations of their low resilience include lashing out with violent "White rage" that can lead to mass murders, increasing rates of suicide, behavioral health issues, and substance use disorders. The strength of their resilience has weakened over time.

"Dudes" and "dudettes" fail to recognize the harms of rudimentary ways of thinking and remain separate and distinct from real men and women who don't subscribe to delusional thinking.

"Dudeism" doesn't have to be a permanent state of being.

Many "dudes" and "dudettes" possess the capacity to decide to depart from their "dudeish" ways by choosing to follow an enlightened path. Unfortunately, many "dudes" and "dudettes" prefer to embrace "Dudeism," rejecting the enlightening wisdom of manhood and womanhood.

According to the American Foundation for Suicide Prevention, White males accounted for nearly 70-percent of all suicide deaths in 2017. A jarring fact since White males are only 30-percent of the American population and enjoy the benefits of White privilege.

Further, the opioid epidemic has primarily ravaged low-income White communities. This outcome is ironic because racist practices in American health care preferentially provide White people with access to higher quality interventions. A common strategy that typically results in better clinical outcomes for White people.

When the premiere "high quality" pain management intervention known as opioids arrived on the scene, White people were the primary recipients. The American health care ecosystem prescribed people of color less potent alternatives. When people of color engage the American health care ecosystem, they are usually viewed as having a higher threshold for pain.

They are often directed to "tough it out" when they share pain management concerns with clinical care teams. When engaging the American health care ecosystem, people of color often have their concerns dismissed and endure condescending attitudes and communications.

Within in-patient or nursing home environments, people of color often witness the needs of White patients prioritized over their own.

With COVID-19, the racist practice of people of color enduring restricted or delayed access to health care interventions reared its ugly head once again. While the racial disparities in COVID-19 infection and mortality rates stand as a broad manifestation of the pervasiveness of this crisis, the Facebook Live video of Dr. Susan Moore is an individual manifestation of this crisis.

Dr. Susan Moore, a physician in Indiana, got infected with COVID-19 and decided to record and share a video of her encounter with the American health care ecosystem. Reporting from a hospital bed with an oxygen tube in her nose, she shared details of her harrowing experience with a clinical team that refused to take her concerns seriously.

Even though she was a physician, they couldn't see past her "Blackness." She died two weeks after sharing the video detailing her harrowing experience.

When COVID-19 vaccines became available, the crisis reared its ugly head once again.

Despite evidence to the contrary, many mass media outlets chose to scapegoat the Tuskegee Syphilis experiment as the leading cause of Black hesitancy to receiving vaccines. They claimed it was why there was a glaring disparity in vaccination rates between White people and Black people.

In reality, inequitable access to vaccines is the actual cause of disparities in vaccination rates between White people and Black people. Inequities are enabled by the complexity, digital, and transportation requirements for accessing vaccination sites and vaccine appointments.

Those inequities are pervasive and insidious. Particularly troubling was the emergence of widespread incidences of rich White people preferentially gaining access to COVID-19 vaccines administered at sites in predominantly lower-income Black and Brown communities.

An equally upsetting casualty of the promotion of White supremacy by the American media industrial complex is the chilling effect "White male savior" propaganda has on some males of color and women of any race.

Males of color and women who, if afforded the opportunity, are capable of being the exceptional, empathetic, and resilient visionaries we need leading American institutions.

However, because of Whitewashing, societal norms, centuries of oppression, uninspiring representation in media, and limited direct exposure to viable role models, many exceptional males of color and women of any race never even try to pursue increasingly higher positions of authority.

They often settle for supporting roles.

Scientific research supports the notion that after a person has been beaten down by repeated opposition to their forward progression, they believe they cannot control or change the situation. They tend to lose motivation once they reach that point.

I conducted some "experiments" when I was a child. When I trapped a fly in a jar, I noticed that after bumping its head against the lid in futile attempts to escape, it would eventually accept its fate and stop trying to fly out of the jar even after I removed the lid.

According to American psychologist Martin Seligman, learned helplessness is related to the concept of self-efficacy: the individual's belief in their innate ability to achieve goals.

Scientists building on Seligman's work have been able to ascertain to a certain degree the detrimental effects of learned helplessness on mental and physical well-being. Learned helplessness is linked to increased feelings of stress, depression, and Post Traumatic Stress Disorder (PTSD).

While professional scientists in various contexts have studied the effects of learned helplessness and conditioned thinking enabled by Whitewashing, I believe we have a lot more to learn. We are yet to ascertain the full extent and entirety of the negative externalities of learned helplessness and conditioned thinking enabled by Whitewashing. Those negative externalities are affecting both White people and people of color in America. And around the world.

A negative externality is a cost that individuals, groups, or society bear due to an economic transaction a third party didn't explicitly consent to. According to Investopedia, externalities by nature are generally environmental, such as natural resources or public health.

For example, a negative externality is a business that causes pollution that diminishes people's property values or health in the surrounding area. In that scenario, property owners and residents didn't have a say in the decision made by the business to pollute their neighborhood.

They just get to bear the cost of the harmful decision the business made.

Given the veracity of the crisis mentioned above, I hypothesize that there is a causal link between the rise in suicide deaths, opioid misuse, and the existence of a growing population of mediocre White "dudes" in America.

Mediocre White "dudes" lack the resilience to accept the reality that they are incapable of manifesting the fantasy America fed them about how exceptional they are supposed to be.

A fantasy about the lives they are "entitled" to lead in America.

A fantasy about their "Whiteness."

This inability to accept reality ultimately causes more pain than they can bear and often leads to destructive behavior that results in self-harm or external harm. The root cause of the pain largely remains unacknowledged. And the resulting behavioral health issues persist.

I often wonder if we will ever redesign the American health care ecosystem to address this calamity.

Given current trends and the absence of any intervention, I assume the American health care industrial complex will choose to double down on the status quo. They will remain focused on feeding the beast that's prioritizing incremental change.

Their behavior enables our collective and treacherous journey to a more consolidated, lower-value health care ecosystem that continues to undermine American prosperity.

The foundation of the current global industrial revolution is Science, Technology, Engineering, Art, and Mathematics (STEAM).

Suppose American institutions continue to promote White supremacy. In that case, a construct I further define as the preferential installation of White people—especially males—in positions of authority over better qualified and more capable people of color. <u>In reality, White mediocrity is what those American institutions are advancing</u>.

White mediocrity that will hasten the erosion of American prosperity.

White mediocrity will cause White people to fail in their quest to secure a better future for White people in America.

Advancing White mediocrity will only cause what White people fear most—loss of power, influence, and economic prosperity—to come to pass sooner rather than later.

America and western democracy flourish when American society musters the courage to acknowledge the reality and negative externalities associated with America's sordid past and present-day injustices. But, unfortunately, if current trends persist, it is easy to foresee the minimal influence western democracy will have in the future.

2050 is the year the forecasts have Nigeria overtaking America as the third most populous country globally. India and China will remain in the first two spots. Although the stated bedrock of American democracy is equal opportunity, our nation's founders were mainly "lower born" White people. They were tired of being oppressed by monarchies and aristocracies—the British Empire—that wanted to continue to tax and control their activities in the Americas.

The White settlers in America knew the "powers that be" wouldn't permit them to ascend to the highest levels of authority in the British Empire because of the social class to which they were born. They wanted to change their destiny, so the White settlers banded together, rebelled, and sought to conquer and subjugate America as the land they could call their own. A place where they could exert power and influence for generations to come. American democracy and institutions were established and optimized to ensure that White males, regardless of their competency or socioeconomic status at birth, have resources, a path to generate wealth and ascend to positions of power and authority in American society.

White "dudes" have a rudimentary understanding of the U.S. Constitution and the ideals on which American democracy was established.

White "dudes" feel threatened by efforts to extend the promise of equal opportunity to males of color and females of any race. I view this manifestation of an inherent fear of the "other" as a tacit acknowledgment by White dudes that they can only excel when males of color and females of any race are disadvantaged from fairly competing for the same opportunities.

After enduring several instances of being referred to as a dude by my wife, Bolanle, I created the construct of a "dude" representing an underdeveloped male that has yet to attain the standard for what a real man should be. She would admonish me from a place of love and a desire not to be slanderous. Often exasperatedly referring to me as a dude when my quirks became overwhelming or my patriarchal tendencies flared up. Usually, only after I pushed her to the brink.

Thankfully those instances have materially reduced over the years.

Her admonishment cut deep and challenged me.

I eventually realized that <u>I owed it to myself and my legacy to be a better man</u>.

A man I could be proud of all the time.

A man my wife, children, and loved ones could be proud of all the time.

A man of substance and character.

A man committed to leaving his house, family, nation, and the world a better place.

While I have attained a certain level of enlightenment, I'll admit I'm still a work in progress. Unfortunately, too many males haven't achieved a meaningful level of refinement, and the "dudes" among them continue to cause irreparable harm to themselves, their families, and their communities. That irreparable harm is rooted in their desire to propagate the oppressive hierarchy of extreme patriarchy.

A hierarchy that favors and elevates males above females simply because of the <u>differences in their genitalia at birth</u>.

Genitalia, not because of any inherent qualities that would cause rational people to default to males always knowing what's best or having the final say.

A "dude's" desire to control a female's right to choose or have agency over when she reproduces is a classic manifestation of a "dude's" desire to have the power to maintain an economic advantage over females. "Dudes" know that they can reduce competition by ensuring that every unplanned conception disadvantages females from equitably competing with them.

When childcare requirements intensify with increases in the number of children in the mix, "dudes" gain more advantage since most households remain constrained by the antiquities of extreme patriarchy. Homes that embrace extreme patriarchy are designed to have females "own" all the domestic responsibilities by default, including childcare responsibilities. "Dudes" are keen to establish extreme patriarchy in their homes as they seek to gain an advantage over the females in their lives.

While it is obvious why a "dude" with a rudimentary understanding of the value of fairness, open competition, and equity would be keen to embrace the philosophies of extreme patriarchy, I remain somewhat perplexed as to why so many females continue to endorse and propagate such extremist views. Such antiquated ideas put females at a disadvantage over the males in their lives and society at large.

A particularly confounding reality is that most White females in America continue to propagate extreme patriarchy in America. They do so through their votes and decision to pander to the egos of mediocre White "dudes."

White females possess the power to tip the scales and enable the election of competent leaders that can implement policies and laws designed to level the playing field for all females. Unfortunately, <u>most White females continue to vote against their socioeconomic interests</u>.

I don't understand all the reasons for the voting patterns of America's population of White females. I assume the decision by most White females to vote against their socioeconomic interests is inspired by their misguided support for the hierarchy of White supremacy. A hierarchy that keeps White females perpetually in a subordinate role to White males.

Even with the rise and fading away of the #metoo movement, most White females continue to vote against their socioeconomic interests.

The White "dude's" tacit acknowledgment that he can only excel when males of color and females of any race are disadvantaged from fairly competing is ironic. The entire construct of White supremacy is that "Whiteness" somehow bestows "superiority." It doesn't.

The reality couldn't be further from the truth.

American democracy has inequitably advanced White males over everyone else since the nation's founding. As such, White male "outperformance" in America when compared to males of color and females of any race is attributable to privileges and advantages enjoyed by White males and not some inherent "superiority" attributable to their "White maleness."

Unfortunately for American society, the "advantage" bestowed on White "dudes" ultimately erodes the excellence, character, and resilience that comes from participating in fair and open competition with all qualified persons without regard for race or gender.

Most White "dudes" were preferentially advanced—and likely lacked the courage to fight and die in American wars—without facing the characteristic elements of natural selection other groups contend with across generations. The bell curve is a common type of distribution for a variable: in this instance, differing racial and gender groups in America. I posit that the bell curve of America's population of White "dudes" skews towards mediocrity, low character, and low resilience.

Racially and gender disadvantaged groups like Black women have a bell curve skewed towards excellence, strong character, and high resilience developed due to the challenges and adversity they had to overcome to survive and advance across generations.

This stark contrast manifested in the reaction, attitude, and follow-up actions pursued by President Trump and Stacey Abrams after losing elections they each claimed were rigged against them.

America and western democracy benefit when our leaders are exceptional, empathetic, and resilient people. Leaders with the character and courage to do right by all Americans regardless of race, gender, religion, or sexual orientation.

White supremacy isn't uniquely American or Anglo-Saxon.

"Whiteness" isn't uniquely toxic.

The fascist Nazi movement and the rise of Adolf Hitler originated in Germany. And the BRIC nations—Brazil, Russia, India, and China—that recently received praise as looming usurpers of America's economy all have sordid histories and are sometimes much worse offenders.

I seriously doubt I would have flourished as a 19-year old Black male immigrant landing in the airport of any BRIC nation in 2002—the year I immigrated to America.

While pursuing my MBA at Stanford University from 2010-to-2012, I had the opportunity to participate in student-organized experience (GER), and immersion (GMIX) trips to Brazil, India, and China. I'm probably never setting foot in Russia. I experienced racism in each of those countries. The overt racism weighed on me after leaving each country.

My most traumatizing experience occurred in Brazil, a White settler nation of mostly Portuguese ancestry. A country where enslaved people from Africa endured one of the most brutal and dehumanizing experiences in any White settler nation during the trans-Atlantic slave trade. A nation where its police force has officially <u>murdered more than 9,000 Black men in the last decade</u>. The real numbers are much higher. Much, much higher.

Brazilian police murder 900 Black men a year.

Brazilian police murder 75 Black men a month.

Brazilian police murder 17 Black men a week.

Brazilian police murder 3 Black men a day.

Brazilian police murder a Black man every 8 hours.

In its manifestations of White supremacy, Brazil remains unsophisticated. Its White ruling class hasn't even decided to embrace fair meritocracy in sports. A transition America made after choosing to integrate sports leagues and teams. The masses compelled the White people. With integration and delivery of more excellent offerings, White people intentionally designed the business models of sports to ensure that White people would still disproportionately profit from the value created in sports dominated by athletes of color.

Brazil's decision not to embrace fair meritocracy in sports ultimately caused its humiliating exit from the 2014 World Cup. A spectacle they hosted with the hopes of showing the world how "White" they were. Unfortunately, their racist decision ignored the obvious reality that more than half of all Brazilians—a nation of more than 200 million people—identify as mixed-race or Black. That fact makes Brazil the White settler nation with the largest mass of surviving descendants of enslaved people from Africa.

While the history and current situation in Brazil is horrendous, there are worse examples in South America. For instance, while Brazil continued to import enslaved people from Africa well into the mid-to-late 1800s, their White European neighbors, from Spain, who settled in Argentina, systematically eradicated their population of enslaved Africans throughout the 1800s. According to historical accounts, from mid-1860 to mid-1870, the President of Argentina, Domingo Faustino Sarmiento, enabled the genocide of most Afro-Argentinean populations using the most barbaric, inhumane, and cruel tactics at the time.

While COVID-19 has decimated Black households in America, the devastation of the COVID-19 pandemic on the Black community in Brazil has been equally bad and much worse in specific scenarios.

In 2020 as the coronavirus pandemic wore on and rates of infection and death rose, President Bolsonaro of Brazil and President Trump seemed to hit it off. As the year wore on, they appeared to be comparing notes and exchanging strategies on denying the existence of the devastating impact of COVID-19 on communities of color in their respective countries.

As an unabashed White "dude," President Trump is the paragon of White mediocrity and a vocal promoter of primal White supremacy^{TM}. His political ascent unapologetically centered on the promotion of primal White supremacy^{TM}.

He elicited a passionate and fanatical response from his supporters. They are the primary beneficiaries of American institutions designed to promote White supremacy.

Unfortunately for the masses that passionately follow President Trump, while he was presenting himself as fighting to advance the economic interests of primal White supremacists™, the majority of his Presidency and Administration was devoted to causes and initiatives that primarily benefited elitist White supremacists™.

White supremacy is designed to advantage White people.

It may appear illogical to expect most White Americans, driven by self-interest and a desire to secure a better future for their White descendants, to vote against a platform that unapologetically commits to upholding White people above everyone else.

President Trump's platform promised to continue to provide White people with preferential access to economic opportunities and positions of power and authority.

Motivated by base instincts of self-preservation, it might appear logical and even alluring for most White people to promote White supremacy as a means of ensuring the advancement of their White descendants.

However, that argument falls apart for me when I consider that for all that has been done to preferentially advance mediocre White "dudes" and "dudettes" above more capable people of color, America continues to fall behind. Many White people, mainly those with no college education or advanced technical skills, continue to hurt.

Substance abuse.

Suicide deaths.

Depression.

Alcoholism.

Low wages.

Job loss.

Intimate partner violence, etcetera.

Mediocrity typically propagates mediocrity.

In the presence of excellence, the shortcomings of mediocre people are readily apparent. Mediocre people lack the resilience to witness their weaknesses contrasted against the talent of exceptional "subordinates." When mediocre people ascend to positions of authority, they resist exceptional people and seek to eliminate peers and subordinates they perceive will illuminate their shortcomings.

Societies that systematically disenfranchise or murder people—based on their skin color or socioeconomic status—capable of being the exceptional, empathetic, and visionary leaders institutions need, will always contend with moral decay and economic malaise.

White supremacists seeking to establish a system of apartheid in America need to look no further than present-day Brazil for a snapshot of what their vision for American society will resemble when White people decline to less than 50-percent of the American population in the mid-2040s.

An apartheid state is a nation dominated politically, socially, and economically by its minority White population.

White supremacists often complain about the presence and proportion of people of color in America.

They assume a historical "Whitening" of America would have improved the life outcomes of White people.

It wouldn't have.

They should examine Argentina's history and current situation to catch a glimpse of what that dystopian fantasy would likely manifest in America.

In reality, the best way to ensure the success of White people in America is to establish a democracy that works for all Americans.

A reimagined American democracy empowered to promote excellence, empathy, and a fair meritocracy above the propagation of White mediocrity.

That new, equitable, merit-based American democracy will maximize everyone's opportunities.

It will ensure that the most exceptional and empathetic individuals rise to positions of authority in American institutions and across American society.

"Prejudice is an emotional commitment to ignorance."
— Nathan Rutstein

The American Health Care Ecosystem Isn't Broken

"In a chronically leaking boat, energy devoted to changing vessels is more productive than energy devoted to patching leaks."
— Warren Buffett

Pondering what it would take to invent an American health care ecosystem that works for all Americans has caused me to internalize three quotes:

1. "Each system is perfectly designed to give you exactly what you are getting today." — W. Edwards Deming
2. "Edison's electric light did not come about from the continuous improvement of the candle." — Oren Harari.
3. "Truth—or, more precisely, an accurate understanding of reality—is the essential foundation for any good outcome." — Ray Dalio

Collectively, these three quotes inspire me to think boldly while also recognizing that entrenched forces are allergic to the truth and committed to maintaining the status quo. Those same forces are pretty adept at investing in incremental change that won't make a difference in the long run. As such, with every bold idea or plan for paradigm-shifting change, I identify incumbent forces incentivized to oppose paradigm-shifting change while building coalitions of support to counter predictable attacks and help actualize the changes we collectively seek.

I've embraced the reality that the current American health care ecosystem isn't "damaged" or in need of repair, like a bicycle with a bent wheel would be considered damaged and in need of a replacement wheel to repair it. Neither is the American health care ecosystem "broken" and in need of a repair, like a bicycle with a broken gear shift would be considered broken and in need of a repair. A repair that would return the bicycle's operating system that is controlled by the gear shift back to its original, functioning design.

Instead, <u>the American health care "system" is functioning as designed</u>—complex, expensive, and inequitable.

Given the pervasiveness of issues that plague health care consumers within certain racial groups and income brackets, among other things, I've embraced the reality that the American health care ecosystem functions as designed and isn't broken, damaged, or in need of repair.

Instead, the American health care ecosystem needs to be reimagined and redesigned with essential stakeholders invited to the decision-making table first. This approach to reform would be a seismic shift from current reform efforts that cede advantage to powerful incumbent stakeholders who become more potent after each health reform cycle. At the same time, essential groups like consumers and front-line workers continue to see their potency eroded.

While I wouldn't consider the internal combustion engine (ICE) ecosystem "damaged" or "broken," those of us who believe in science have come to acknowledge the urgent need to innovate and scale climate-friendly alternative ecosystems.

Fortunately, the implementation of regulatory and financial incentives catalyzed the creation and growth of a valuable electric car ecosystem that barely relies on fossil fuels.

The approach to developing alternatives to fossil-fueled vehicles is attractive. We should adopt it for the American health care industry. Further exploration of the evolution of the American transportation industry and the varied alternative modes of transportation contained within it could serve as an example of how the structure, delivery, and payments within a reimagined American health care ecosystem could work.

Everyone can't afford to drive a complicated, high-maintenance, luxury car to move from point A to B. Simpler and cheaper cars, mass transit options, bicycle lanes, and sidewalks ensure that transitioning from point A to B is accessible and affordable for most of the people in America. While the American transportation industry isn't a paragon of excellence or innovation by any stretch of the imagination, it still manages to serve more Americans than the American health care industry satisfactorily.

Innovative new entrants like Tesla have led our ongoing transition from ICE-powered automobiles to fully electric alternatives. Similarly, I posit that innovative new entrants are our best chance to realize the American health care ecosystem we need: simple, affordable, and equitable.

Influential incumbent stakeholders across the American health care industry are unlikely to lead us to the "Promised Land" and deliver the re-imagined American health care ecosystem we need. History shows that incumbents are incentivized to retain and protect accumulated power instead of supporting innovation that may adversely impact their invested assets. A reality that is manifest in the outcomes of health reform efforts attempted in the last several decades.

Incumbents' assets typically serve as a moat and help to preserve current power dynamics. The fee-for-service transaction ecosystem, institutional knowledge, and legacy technology systems that currently power American health care serves as foundational elements of the moat that continues to advantage incumbents and disadvantage innovative new entrants and would-be disruptors.

I concluded that the American health care "system" is functioning as designed after spending the last year holed up in my house because of the COVID-19 pandemic. The time I spent quarantining allowed me to reflect on my almost twenty years of experience as an advisor, operator, investor, and civil servant. My experience using my knowledge of the American health care industry to empower different stakeholder groups I supported over the years.

I believe that achieving better health outcomes for all Americans and less harmful fiscal results for taxpayers will require more than any of the current or proposed reforms that have the nation <u>hurtling towards a seven trillion dollar American health care ecosystem by 2030</u>.

A "system" I anticipate will be increasingly consolidated.

A "system" that offers less.

A "system" that costs us more.

A "system" accelerating the erosion of America's comparative advantage in the domestic production of goods and services.

Unlike most costs, American society bears American health care costs. Unreasonably high health care costs adversely impact all companies and people who choose to call America home. American health care costs, prices, and spending undermine America's prosperity and, ultimately, its influence worldwide. The adverse impact typically manifests as significant liabilities on corporate balance sheets, shrinking disposable income in consumer wallets, stagnating wages, declining investment in other critical services, and increasing domestic production costs.

As American health care spending eclipses twenty percent of America's Gross Domestic Product (GDP) and races towards twenty-two percent of America's GDP by 2030, the American health care industry continues to attract more talent and resources to support its growth. This trend is very concerning not only because of the significant concentration of the American economy on an industry with so much waste but also because of the opportunity cost of the talent and resources seeking to profit from the bloated American health care industry. Instead of deploying additional talent and resources to support innovation and growth in other essential sectors, the overinvestment of talent and resources to support wasteful spending across the American health care industry continues to scale.

Globalization and automation continue to decimate other industries where America lacks a comparative advantage in domestic production. Ironically partly due to unreasonably high health care costs, prices, and spending. However, American health care job growth has steadily increased and supported most local economies because legal and regulatory constraints keep most health care jobs and investment dollars in local economies.

Evaluating our current realities reminds me of what some of my former economics professors used to say, "Protectionism isn't a sustainable long-term strategy for growth or economic development." At Howard, Cyril Hunte, Haydar Kurban, and Bill Spriggs. And at Stanford, Renee Bowen.

Consider for a moment where America would be if it didn't abolish slavery and instead recommitted to exploiting unpaid labor of enslaved people. Oh wait, it is currently manifesting as inequitable mass incarceration of Black and Brown people. Exacerbating this crisis are the inequities in institutional investment in American males of color and females of all races. How much worse off would those local economies be today if America stuck with labor-intensive approaches to cotton production and other low-value commodities that America heavily subsidizes today?

Before the industrial revolutions that transformed modern society, most local economies in America were living fat and happy off the economic rents that the unpaid labor of enslaved people afforded them. Economic rents are distinct from revenue and profit attainable in a competitive market because it represents financial gain above what is economically and socially necessary. As such, I imagine most local economies were likely resistant to adopting innovative solutions they viewed as being "too disruptive" to the status quo.

To clarify, I am in no way, shape, or form comparing slavery or the Trans-Atlantic slave trade to the market dynamics of the American health care industry. However, because it is easier for incumbents, new entrants, and other stakeholders to extract economic rents by enabling the status quo, they choose to take the easier path.

Enabling the status quo might seem more prudent in the short run. However, incumbents, new entrants, and other stakeholders that complicity endorse the status quo are in for a rude awakening in the long run.

The cohort I anticipate will suffer the most from the eventual fallout will be the local economies primarily dependent on extracting economic rents from their lower-value, local health care ecosystems. Those health care ecosystems lack inherent comparative advantage in the delivery of value-based care and payments.

Incumbents, new entrants, and other stakeholders that primarily pursue paradigm-shifting, higher-value, and globally relevant health care innovation would better serve American society.

According to the United States Bureau of Labor, one out of every nine jobs in America directly supports the American health care industry. A quarter or more of all American jobs are directly or indirectly linked to the American health care industry.

While job growth is desirable, the opportunity cost of health care job growth is that America continues to fall further behind in developing globally relevant assets and technology.

While incumbent stakeholders and many new entrants are eager to seek more economic rents from the American health care industry, the goods and services they are developing and delivering in exchange for those economic rents have limited value across the globe.

Market failures lead to a rise in economic rents because competitive markets are designed to drive down prices and minimize economic rent-seeking behavior.

When companies are enticed by the opportunity to extract economic rents from the American health care industry, scarce software engineering talent is deployed to advance the evolution of Artificial Intelligence (AI), Machine Learning (ML), and other emerging technologies. Those efforts are focused on automating and enhancing overly complicated American health care ecosystem transactions.

I posit that scarce technical talent dedicated to advancing the byzantine idiosyncrasies of the American health care industry can deliver more intrinsic, globally relevant value if deployed to tackle problems associated with inherently complicated issues. Such talent could resolve complicated calamities like climate change, suicide, domestic abuse, income inequality, poverty, human trafficking, etcetera.

Referencing a joke from the 1967 comic strip Wizard of Id, "Remember the golden rule! What's that? Whoever has the gold makes the rules!" I surmise that the rest of the world continues to invest talent and resources to support "innovation" in the American health care industry because America is currently the largest economy and health care market in the world.

Incentives cause most specialized human talent to support activities that result in the most significant economic rents, not activities that result in the most incredible intrinsic value to the general population.

As a self-motivated problem solver and health care futurist, the last year has been particularly challenging for me to endure. I put "pen to paper" (Actually typed directly into a computer. I'm a millennial) to begin the work of writing this book on the day we set aside to honor the birth and legacy of Reverend Dr. Martin Luther King Jr. (MLK).

This MLK day is unlike any of the ones that preceded it since it is occurring as the nation reels from a recent violent attack on the U.S. Capitol by an insurrectionist mob enraged by the outcome of the 2020 presidential election.

Later that week, we inaugurated President Biden and Vice President Harris. They had a swearing-in ceremony conducted with sparse crowds under the protection of the police, federal law enforcement, and more than 20,000 National Guard troops. Forces that converted downtown

Washington D.C. to what I assume the green zone of a war-torn "developing nation" would resemble.

That imagery is a far cry from where I imagine Reverend Dr. Martin Luther King Jr. would have hoped we would be as a nation pursuing a perfect union almost 60 years after his "I have a dream" speech. He delivered his speech on the steps of the Lincoln Memorial during the March on Washington for Jobs and Freedom.

The anticipated mob violence in protest of the inauguration of President Biden and Vice President Harris wasn't the only reason large cheering crowds didn't manifest for the swearing-in ceremony of a Presidential ticket that garnered the most votes in American history. Rather, equally concerning was the risk of assembling large crowds during a deadly pandemic that had claimed almost half a million American lives by the inauguration of President Biden and Vice President Harris.

Like the violent riots, subsequent damage, and deaths that occurred on January 6, 2021, we could have avoided the extensive harm caused by the COVID-19 pandemic if we had competent leaders that recognized the severity of the looming challenges and took requisite action.

While many sought to sensationalize the events of January 6, 2021, as a failed coup attempt, I saw it very differently since I was born and raised in Nigeria, a nation that experienced several failed and successful coup d'état's when I lived there.

I heard about the successful 1983 military coup d'état led by Major-General Muhammadu Buhari. He is the current "democratically elected" President of Nigeria. I used air quotes because the British Empire designed their colonies to fail as independent nations. The British Empire didn't construct its colonies to thrive as functioning democracies. Buhari is as democratically elected as Putin is. It was his turn. It is Tinubu's turn next. Babangida is the godfather of them all. Babangida the evil genius: a well-earned moniker.

I witnessed the adverse effects of the tyrannical rule of military dictators like General Ibrahim Badamosi Babangida (IBB) and General Sani Abacha. General Abacha was so uncouth. So ruthless. Easily the worst of the lot.

I can't fathom America ever experiencing an actual coup attempt.

Or a successful coup d'état.

Its established institutions and systems of checks and balances will prevent that.

For that to remain true, America's institutions must check and balance each other.

Any weakened democracy can collapse.

Any weakened democracy can become subjected to authoritarian rule.

As I explained (very liberal use of the word) to former Secretary of State Condoleezza Rice during a sidebar conversation after a class she taught in 2010, Nigeria is an oligarchy masquerading as a democracy. The course was the Global Context of Management course she co-taught with Professor Bill Barnett, and the case discussion in class that day was on the Dubai Ports controversy. As she expressed optimism for what the Administration of recently installed President Goodluck Johnathan (GEJ) would do to promote peace and prosperity while advancing western democracy in the region, I advised her to lower her expectations.

Even though I considered it a sign of progress that Nigerian oligarchs allowed a peaceful civilian transition after President Yar'Adua died, Nigerian institutions are currently incapable of enabling a well-functioning democracy. There were concerns about another coup d'état transpiring because President Yar'Adua from a different tribe didn't get to serve his full term. Prosperous nations need a well-functioning democracy with competent leaders who are empowered to enact the people's will or put the country on a path to prosperity.

In our conversation, I posited that achieving widespread prosperity for Nigeria and most of its indigenes wasn't likely on the current path. Nigeria needs to establish an empathetic form of market-oriented benevolent autocracy. Leaders in the market-oriented benevolent autocracy would establish a viable, multi-decade economic development plan. That viable, multi-decade economic development plan would enable and scale Nigerian prosperity. An empathetic market-oriented benevolent autocracy is a better alternative to the socioeconomic malaise caused by the folly and greed of the Nigerian oligarchy.

I proffered that the market-oriented benevolent autocrats would focus on developing the nation's institutions and laying a foundation for a viable, well-functioning democracy to assume power once the country is on an established path to prosperity.

I shared that I thought it was prudent for African and western watchdogs to be engaged to keep the market-oriented benevolent autocrats focused on the mission. She indulged me for a few minutes longer. We didn't have any other discourse until the day before my MBA graduation ceremony in 2012. I met with her (in her Hoover tower office) to solicit her perspective on accelerating my career, establishing my paths to power, and constructing my American political ideology.

During our discussion, I shared some concerns I had about the inherent harms of the rhetoric and actions of the Tea Party (birther) movement. Concerns about the inherent harms of the birther movement on American political discourse and civility more broadly. She dismissed my concerns by explaining that despite the antics of the birther movement, the Republican Party had succeeded in nominating capable Republicans like Mitt Romney and Paul Ryan to lead the presidential ticket in 2012.

While a well-functioning democracy is ideal, in a nation where its oligarchs continue to exchange the nation's collective birthright for the proverbial "bowl of porridge," absent any intervention, Nigeria is already on its way back to being subjected to autocratic rule. I assume Communist China will gain complete control of Nigeria by 2050. It may happen sooner.

2050 is the same year when Nigeria, the largest Black nation in the world, will be the third-largest country globally. Those projections forecast that America will fall to fourth place by 2050.

Consider for a moment how little progress America would make if it had to try and establish its democratic institutions and invest in the nation's infrastructure with a bitterly divided electorate. Now, imagine splintering the electorate into hundreds of factions. Then, imagine those factions spoke different languages, worshipped various "deities," and harbored so much hatred of the "other" that self-mutilation (tribal marks) to signal tribal affiliation (since everyone is Black) was commonplace. How much progress would America make towards establishing democratic institutions or effectively investing in critical infrastructure in such a scenario?

I posit that a well-functioning democracy is a luxury and a privilege. It should manifest in advanced societies with an electorate of predominantly informed critical thinkers who can distinguish between fact and fiction. For democracy to shine, the majority of a nation's population must achieve that level of enlightenment. Till then, efforts should focus on establishing equitable and commendable legislative, judicial, and executive institutions by any means necessary.

Celebrating the illusion of a well-functioning democracy while oligarchs rule may not be the best approach to take when attempting to put fragmented communities forcibly conjoined by colonialism on a path to prosperity.

I primarily viewed the insurrectionist mob that attacked the U.S. Capitol akin to a violent tantrum thrown by petulant adults spoiled as children.

Those petulant adults are routinely shielded from negative consequences by American institutions. They are accustomed to having things go their way.

As I watched the melee unfold on television, I was reminded of a recent mini-tantrum our 3-year old, Arielle, threw. She threw a mini-tantrum the first time we played the board game chutes and ladders with her 5-year old sister, Briella. The mini-tantrum erupted after her "roll of the dice" (the version we have has a wheel with a spinning arrow) landed her playing token on the longest slide near the finish line. The slide she landed on moved her playing token back to the last place, terminating in an area close to the starting line.

As she started throwing a fit and yelling, "I don't wanna go down the slide," she attempted to flip the board. I stopped her and reminded her that we were all playing by the same rules and that just because she had a setback, she shouldn't give up or throw a fit. After she calmed down, she kept playing and ultimately came in second place after Briella won the game. I didn't throw the game; they outplayed me. Lucky spins.

Unfortunately for western democracy, the insurrectionist mob that attacked the U.S. Capitol Building lacked responsible supervision and was invited to Washington D.C. by President Trump, who refused to acknowledge he lost the 2020 election. Instead, he threw a tantrum and pursued several futile attempts to try and get his way by subverting the will of most Americans.

The insurrectionist mob consisted of a diverse cohort of mostly White "dudes" like the "horn guy" (QAnon Shaman), an out-of-work Navy veteran who lived with his mother after being evicted for failing to pay his rent. Also in the crowd were White "dudettes" like the "real estate lady" who could afford to fly into D.C. on a private charter. The socioeconomic diversity of the White "dudes" and "dudettes" that participated in the January 6, 2021 mob violence highlighted that Trumpism is about more than just securing economic advantage for low-income, downtrodden, low-skilled White people.

As the events of that fateful day unfolded, I reflected on Stacey Abrams' actions after losing the race to become Georgia's governor in 2018. That election was fraught with allegations that the eventual winner, Brian Kemp, was proactively suppressing the vote of the portion of the electorate more inclined to vote for his opponent, Stacey Abrams. Brian Kemp was Georgia's Secretary of State at the time. He was the White "dude" setting the rules and policies for an election in which he was contesting.

I also attempted to imagine what would have happened in 2016 if President Obama invited a diverse array of primarily Black people to a Washington D.C. rally. A rally to protest and try to subvert Senator Mitch McConnell's decision to block President Obama's nominee for the vacant Supreme Court seat.

Comparing and contrasting the "scandals" and related consequences from the Obama Administration years and the Trump Administration years reminded me—not that I've ever forgotten—that White supremacy continues to thrive across American society.

Finally, choosing to frame the events of January 6, 2021, as a failed coup attempt would be giving President Trump too much credit.

Packing the courts—at all levels—with elitist White supremacists was designed to serve the fascist agenda of laying a foundation for apartheid in America. Not to keep President Trump in office.

Forecasters expect White people to be less than 50-percent of the American population by the mid-2040s.

Suppose a system of apartheid—a nation dominated politically, socially, and economically by the nation's minority White population—is established in America by the mid-2040s. In that case, American society is likely to have devolved into a country similar to present-day Brazil.

With its sordid history, Brazil is the White settler nation with the largest population of descendants of formerly enslaved people from Africa.

More than half of Brazil's population of 200 million people identifies as mixed-race or Black. The rest of its people mostly descended from White European settlers.

Brazil has notoriously underinvested in its communities of color. It continues to torture, oppress, and exploit its communities of color.

Brazil neglects its communities of color. A decision that leads to devastating racial disparities in income, health, and overall life outcomes for the people of color that live in Brazil.

When a significant proportion of any society is disenfranchised based on the color of their skin, their ethnicity, or socioeconomic status at birth, such a society is bound to be morally reprehensible and suffer from economic malaise.

I think the ulterior motive behind President Trump's claims of election fraud is a continued desire to exploit his political fundraising prowess. His claims also serve as a pretext for more stringent voter suppression laws and help him retain power over the Republican Party and its loyal base of primal White supremacists.

President Trump is a showman and a capitalist obsessed with attention.

He is a White "dude" conditioned to seek new ways to keep eyeballs on his theatrics and coffers full of cash.

All that aside, I acknowledge that the tantrum thrown by the insurrectionist mob for the world to see was an unsettling assault on America's citadel of democracy. It saddens me to think about how the propaganda machine of authoritarian regimes and fascists worldwide will use the televised imagery and violence of January 6, 2021, to undermine democracy. It remains one of the least explored negative externalities from that fateful day.

I do think President Trump lived up to his notorious classification as a Useful Idiot (UI), though. The Return on Investment (ROI) to the "pro-life" voting bloc and Vladimir Putin was more significant than either could've imagined when they decided to get in bed with Trumpism.

But like fish that had turned, once he lost the 2020 presidential election and ultimately incited a riotous mob to intimidate Congress, he was deemed to have passed his expiration date and needed to be tossed in the trash. I assume until he can reprise his role as a UI.

Classifying the attack on the U.S. Capitol as a coup attempt, even a poorly planned one, is merely another manifestation of American mediocrity.

Like most established institutions in America, the American health care industrial complex is optimized to serve the needs of a subset of the American population. That service is typically delivered at the expense of less wealthy people of color in American society.

From the prison industrial complex to the law enforcement industrial complex and the higher education industrial complex, etcetera, American institutions were primarily established on a foundation of White supremacy.

Viewing current events through the lens of my lived experiences provides greater illumination. I further define a foundation of White supremacy as a mindset that seeks to promote a hierarchical order with wealthy, White Anglo-Saxon Protestant (WASP) males at the top of the hierarchy and low-income Black women at the very bottom of the hierarchy.

American institutions are increasingly optimized to serve this hierarchy preferentially. Those same institutions are upholding multi-generational outcomes predetermined by access to economic opportunity. Results are influenced by the psychological safety accessible to each group based on their position in that hierarchy.

While the majority of the electorate isn't at the very top of the hierarchical order propagated by White supremacy, they aren't at the very bottom either. Many are seemingly all too willing to continue to uphold, instead of disrupting, the hierarchy of White supremacy and the negative externalities it inflicts on American society.

Most groups will never make it to the very top of the hierarchy upheld by White supremacy. The apex predator will eventually attack "lower-ranked" groups. White females. Asians. Hispanics. LGBTQ etcetera.

Members of the electorate that aren't at the very bottom of the hierarchy often take turns oppressing groups "ranked lower" in the hierarchy. Too many Americans primarily don't mobilize to take action against injustice until it is their turn to be vilified directly or indirectly by the activities of the apex predator.

Mediocre White "dudes," especially the wealthy ones, elevated to positions of authority, are the apex predators dwelling near the top of the hierarchy of White supremacy. Rep. Matt Gaetz. Tucker Carlson. Those "dudes."

White supremacy in American health care manifests in the health outcomes achieved by different members of the American population it is supposed to serve.

Disparate outcomes in the maternal mortality rates of White and Black women serve as a sordid reminder of the pervasive influence of the hierarchy of White supremacy in the American health care ecosystem. According to the Centers for Disease Control and Prevention (CDC), in 2020, Black women were over three times more likely to die in childbirth than White women.

Black and Brown households in America have mostly shouldered the burden of the devastating impact of COVID-19. The hierarchy rears its ugly head again. Disparities in hospitalization rates, mortality, and vaccination between White people and people of color worsened during the COVID-19 pandemic.

In America, except for Asians, people of color were more than twice as likely to die from COVID-19 as White people. Thinking about what the oppressed have done in the past to call attention to these issues, I'm reminded of the sayings, "talk is cheap" and "actions speak louder than words."

American health care is a highly regulated industry that has historically been very slow to implement any changes. The resulting inertia provides ample opportunities for incumbents to insulate their organizations or respective stakeholder groups against anticipated financial harm from any new policy, regulation, or provision of law.

By continually propagating campaign finance corruption, partisan gerrymandering, and voter suppression laws, any incumbent that is sufficiently threatened by proposed or pending legislation, policy or regulation, can invest resources in efforts to influence the process and likely secure a more favorable outcome.

Suffice to say, "All's fair in love, war, and health reform" seems to be the attitude of American health care industry stakeholders. Current campaign finance rules enable capitalistic stakeholders. Laws they helped write and lobbied to get implemented. They view financial contributions to secure a favorable regulatory or policy outcome like an investment in any other asset the stakeholder expects would provide it with a competitive advantage or a financial return.

As demonstrated by prolific influencers in the pharmaceutical industry, the returns they've earned on their investment in lobbying deliver an estimated 15-to-1 ratio compared to their investment in research and development activities to create new therapeutics.

Although with significant taxpayer-funded government resources and appropriations, the pharmaceutical stakeholder group delivered life-saving vaccines in record time to curtail the loss of life from the COVID-19 pandemic. I suspect that the pharmaceutical industry will be "untouchable" in the next decade or so. Health reform priorities will look elsewhere to curb excessive spending and economic rent-seeking behavior.

Many altruists and health reform luminaries remain incensed at the shenanigans of the pharmaceutical industry. I don't blame them. However, choosing to continue deploying capital while wasting time on ongoing futile attempts is the wrong decision.

Economic rent-seeking stakeholders are fighting to boost their financial situation and maximize shareholder returns.

Economic rent-seeking stakeholders are typically willing to deploy resources at levels similar to amounts they anticipate losing with an unfavorable legislative or policy outcome.

For example, let's assume pharmaceutical industry stakeholders anticipate losing 10 billion dollars in annual profits from the successful implementation of a proposed law, regulation, or policy. They would view it as their fiduciary responsibility to spend up to, or more than—driven by the slippery slope fallacy—10 billion dollars to influence the outcome of the proposed law, regulation, or policy.

That level of financial resource will likely never be available to be used by altruists or health reform luminaries that oppose them.

I posit that to move the needle on American health care reform, altruists and reform advocates should invest most of their time and capital on efforts to reform campaign finance corruption, partisan gerrymandering, and voter suppression laws.

Given current trends and the absence of intervention, in thirty years, I anticipate we will be contending with an American health care industry that is extremely consolidated, with only a handful of payviders dominating regional and local markets across the nation. Payviders are vertically integrated payers and providers. In lay terms: Insurance companies acquiring physician groups and other provider entities.

The resulting regional and national health care ecosystems will function more like regulated utilities—hopefully with price controls—than value-oriented, consumer-centric ecosystems optimized to help patients achieve their desired health and well-being outcomes.

Like how companies that provide electricity or gas to consumers' homes function, I posit that future health care consumers will have increasingly limited choices or agency in where they can seek care.

I typically don't give a lot of faith to long-term predictions.

However, in clear-cut scenarios similar to the devastating path we are on regarding climate change, absent any intervention, American health care markets will devolve into actual monopolies or duopolies. Incumbents like UnitedHealth Group, Anthem, and CVS Health will solidify their market-leading positions. New entrants like Amazon and Walmart will settle on a strategy that scales. Together, these five corporations will control most American health care ecosystems in the future.

While many mocked the failure of Haven, the Joint Venture (JV) effort between Berkshire Hathaway, J.P. Morgan, and Amazon, I assume leaders of those companies had ulterior motives for a JV designed to fail from the onset. Ulterior motives, I think, will become readily apparent in the future.

American health care is designed to serve the hierarchy of White supremacy.

It is capitalistic by nature.

My predictions are a logical outgrowth of where things are today.

Monopolies are the most advanced manifestations of capitalism.

Despite all the delusional chants like "this is not who we are" or "I can't believe this is happening in America," we must not forget that the establishment of our beloved nation was bolstered by the genocide of its indigenous people and enslavement of Africans.

Atrocious acts committed to advance an economic growth agenda designed to exploit people of color and establish American institutions intended primarily to propagate the hierarchy of White supremacy.

That is the uncomfortable truth many White Americans refuse to accept.

They didn't fall from the sky.

They descended from the same Americans that committed those historical atrocities. Their ancestors benefited alongside the ones that committed the barbaric acts.

Jim Crow laws, the Chinese Exclusion Act, Japanese-American internment camps, and Operation Wetback serve as sordid 19th and 20th-century reminders of what American institutions are capable of "legalizing" to continue to propagate White supremacy in American society.

In 2021, how are caricatures of Native Americans still appearing on official state flags and as sports team names and mascots? I find it unbelievably abhorrent that the descendants of the indigenous owners—unless they wiped out whoever claimed the land first—of the landmass that is present-day America still have to contend with such indignities.

We are reminded of the unfinished work daily.

Present-day examples of unpunished police brutality, inequitable mass incarceration, unencumbered violent racist attacks, and the "Muslim ban." Other examples include threats or acts of violence by White supremacists not taken seriously by law enforcement, and state-sanctioned institutions that boldly promote bigotry are jarring reminders of the work we have to do.

We are fortunate to no longer live in an America where crowds openly gather and take pictures, jammed together, clamoring, looking for the best angle to watch smoldering and often charred "strange fruit" dangling from trees or overhead bridges.

We still have much to accomplish to establish an American society where race or gender doesn't automatically bestow privilege or disadvantage.

Establishing such a society would be the ultimate manifestation of the American dream.

The pursuit of health is ultimately about achieving optimal life outcomes. Without achieving good or optimal health and well-being outcomes, maximizing other parts of life is near impossible. Achieving excellent or optimal health is the foundation of what makes everything else possible.

I'm encouraged by the expanded adoption of innovative technology and services designed to aid the delivery of care during the COVID-19 pandemic.

However, I remain concerned that the adoption rate will slow or even reverse course once the government lifts social distancing and indoor activity restrictions.

The American health care industrial complex is adept at creating a lot of activity without making any real progress against stated value-creation objectives.

Absent any intervention, the COVID-19 pandemic won't be a turning point for cancer metastasizing at the intersection of White supremacy and American health care.

COVID-19 will ultimately serve as the latest excuse for the American health care industry to become more complex, expensive, and inequitable.

The current American health care ecosystem is designed to encourage patient encounters to occur in the buildings where their clinical care teams work.

The current design allows hospital-centric health systems and owners of those buildings to generate additional revenue by requiring patients to go into those buildings to receive care.

Even when a virtual visit would suffice.

Ancillary clinical services.

Facility fees included in patient's bills

Parking fees that sometimes exceed provider encounter copays.

Food and beverages purchased on the premises.

These line items help boost the top and bottom lines of the increasingly hospital-centric buildings that facilitate most patient's encounters with their clinical care teams.

To create a consumer-centric American health care ecosystem that is simple, affordable, and equitable, we must embrace the evolution of the American health care ecosystem.

An evolved American health care ecosystem is virtual-first, technology-enabled, home-centric, and powered by value-based care and payment infrastructure.

An ecosystem that isn't reliant on legacy fee-for-service reimbursement infrastructure and annual contracting lifecycles.

For America to maximize its domestic and global potential, we must redesign the American health care ecosystem to work for all Americans.

We must rein in American health care costs, prices, and spending.

I remain hopeful that the looming economic destruction and ongoing deterioration of American health outcomes associated with enabling the status quo will serve as a burning platform for America to pursue paradigm-shifting change.

An alternative path to the one we are currently on.

A current path primarily pursuing incremental tweaks.

A current path keeping us on a perilous health reform journey to mediocrity.

Overview of the American Health Care Cartel

"If you don't have a seat at the table, you're probably on the menu. Washington works for those who have power. And no one gives up power easily, no one."
– Senator Elizabeth Warren

Cartels are a group of market stakeholders perceived to be independent but, in reality, are typically in cahoots to grow their collective profits and dominate their market. Operating in the same or closely related businesses, American health care cartel members function as an alliance of rivals.

A rivalry that often culminates in an eagerness to celebrate the excoriation or demise of other American health care cartel members. Excoriation and demise often create opportunities for the "unscathed" to capture revenue and profits lost by excoriated or defunct American health care cartel members.

American antitrust laws exist, and cartels are supposed to be illegal due to their inherently adverse impact on consumers.

Unfortunately for the American health care consumer, some legislators, large employers, and mass media outlets are celebrated but often covert members of the American health care cartel.

Primarily functioning as guardians of the status quo, these American health care cartel members are gatekeepers that ensure all attempts at health reform result in ever-increasing prices and spending on low-value medical care or related infrastructure. A secondary purpose of these American health care cartel members is to serve as fake health reform allies.

Exacerbating the calamity at the intersection of White supremacy and American health care is the negative externality of bloated health care spending. This excessive health care spending results in chronic underinvestment in other essential services like public health, nutrition, social supports, education, science, arts, and civics.

American health care ecosystems are local. As such, some legislators are incentivized to pad as much "health care" funding into government budgets as they can. Padded budgets designed to fund medical care infrastructure in their home state, congressional district, or county.

With shovels in hand and grin's on their faces, some legislators proudly pose for photo opportunities at the groundbreaking of another low-value capital project expansion of the local hospital-centric health system or academic medical center. This capital allocation strategy is primarily designed to support local construction jobs and related services. Building construction, employment, and services that accrue little value to health care consumers or taxpayers.

The government contracts and local construction jobs enabled in the fund flows mentioned above typically represent a return on political campaign contributions from government contractors and employee unions alike.

One of the downsides of the aforementioned economic transactions is that it commits local resources and attention to low-value capital projects while continuing to underinvest in other critical services considered social drivers of health. Those social drivers of health have a more significant impact on improving local health outcomes.

Some large employers are a tricky bunch and have essentially managed to convince the public that they are also victims of the machinations of the American health care cartel.

Further complicating matters, most of the recent job gains in America link to the health care industry. As such, American health care cartel members also have a seat, and a loud voice, at the large employer table. With their seat at the large employer table, American health care cartel members help enable the continuity of the employer-centric health benefits system.

In addition to corporate and tax advantages associated with employer-centric health benefits, some large employers favor higher prices and health benefit costs because it gives them leverage over their employees.

Some employees feel compelled to remain employed in toxic corporate cultures propagated by their large employers instead of pursuing entrepreneurial ventures capable of eventually usurping the market position of large employers.

Most people who work rely on their employers for access to health benefits. Employers have significant leverage over employees who can't afford to quit or lose their jobs because they don't want to lose access to their preferred provider networks. Also, those types of employees can't afford to pay for health benefit premiums independently. Further complicating matters are the significantly higher health benefit costs associated with pursuing entrepreneurship or small business ownership.

Some mass media outlets have incentives to protect and promote the American health care cartel. Their support often manifests as the pervasive promotion of hospital-centric acute care settings as the preeminent site of care. Mass media outlets traditionally get their "cut" from the numerous paid advertisements for overpriced pharmaceuticals, unproven therapeutics, private Medicare Advantage plans, and other health care products and services they get paid to promote on their platforms.

American health care cartel members prefer to take strategic planning cues from Pablo Escobar. Pablo Escobar was the founder of The *Medellín* Cartel, which operated from 1972 to 1993. While taking notes from Pablo Escobar, American health care cartel members willfully ignore Adam Smith.

Adam Smith, regarded as the father of modern economics, wrote The Wealth of Nations, a time-tested book published in 1776. In The Wealth of Nations, Adam Smith raised alarms on the perils of monopolies and promoted the benefits of competitive markets. Benefits he posited would accrue to consumers, societies, nations, and the world.

American health care cartel members lack the leadership excellence and creative vision to manifest paradigm-shifting innovation. They have become adept at establishing pseudo-monopolies and currying favor from the "invisible hand" that steers the "free markets."

In an ideal world, Americans would have legislators who put the fiscal and societal needs of all American's first, large employers who empower their employees with influential seats at the decision-making table, and a mass media ecosystem focused on ensuring the general public is well-informed and aware of the root causes of the market failures that plague American society.

Unfortunately, that ideal world is unlikely to materialize unless we successfully reform campaign finance corruption, partisan gerrymandering, and voter suppression laws.

The underlying business model of medical service delivery that underpins the American health care ecosystem is relatively straightforward. When boiled down, the business model of medical service delivery is essentially matching stakeholders (consumers) who need medical services with stakeholders (providers) capable of delivering the services they need.

Like every other good or service procured, once matched, agreements are subsequently executed between the consumer and the provider to govern the terms of engagement. In an ideal scenario, each stakeholder honors their end of the bargain.

Unfortunately for the health care consumer, the American health care ecosystem is riddled with armies of intermediaries and low-value interlopers conjuring niche approaches designed to extract economic rents from the bloated American health care ecosystem.

The American health care cartel obfuscates what should otherwise be a direct contracting relationship between consumers and providers. Instead, it enables the current approach, which keeps prices and spending high while restricting competition.

While there are many known and veiled members of the American health care cartel, the four primary American health care cartel members are:

1. **Purchasers** (employers, government, etcetera),
2. **Payers** (insurers, public or private insurance agencies, etcetera),
3. **Providers** (hospital-centric health systems, nursing homes, assisted living facilities, dialysis centers, and hospital trade associations, etcetera), and
4. **Producers** (suppliers of pharmaceuticals, esoteric knowledge, information technology, medical equipment and devices, etcetera)

Although the underlying business model of medical service delivery is relatively straightforward, the flow of funds is very complex, opaque, and convoluted. The complexity and opacity of the fee-for-service transaction ecosystem enable the covert flow of funds between American health care cartel members. It remains one of the primary reasons that simplifying or reducing the transaction costs associated with facilitating health care fund flows has been unbelievably challenging to actualize.

Since fee-for-service contracts and transactions are designed to be complicated to execute, producers capable of enabling such complex transactions position themselves to command higher prices for their services.

When competition attempts to drive prices down, American health care cartel members repel new entrants or "slow-walk" the adoption of innovative new approaches until incumbent producers can deliver the same capability in a less "disruptive" manner.

Alternate tactics used include efforts by American health care cartel members to acquire the new entrants and implement post-acquisition integration strategies that quell any attempts to disrupt the status quo.

One of the more sinister tactics utilized by American health care cartel members is regulatory or technical levers used to frustrate any innovative new entrants who seek to disrupt the status quo.

Regulatory approaches usually result in the layering-on of unnecessarily cumbersome requirements incumbents can best meet or technical integration requirements that significantly increase the costs of implementing paradigm-shifting innovative solutions.

The additional cost and complexity of the approach mentioned above to adopting new, innovative solutions have historically eliminated the opportunity to simplify the flow of funds or reduce transaction costs.

Complexity is the enemy of transparency. Transparency is what American health care fund flows and transactions need if we ever hope to simplify and reduce unnecessary spending.

Other American health care cartel members like payers and providers are also incentivized to aggregate and retain information on complex and opaque fee-for-service transactions. This tactic employed by payers and providers is usually to build a proprietary data moat to gain a negotiating advantage when establishing hundreds of mostly annual contracts with other American health care cartel members.

American health care cartel members also use their proprietary knowledge of the complex fee-for-service fund flow and transaction information to extract as much value from their interactions with other American health care ecosystem stakeholders. American health care cartel members are especially adept at using this information asymmetry to their advantage during their interactions with consumers.

Unfortunately, health care consumers have limited insight into the complex and opaque fund flows, transactions, alternative pathways, or price discrepancies. They are typically ill-equipped to be on equal footing or have the advantage when interacting with American health care cartel members.

Although severely disadvantaged, health care consumers pay into American health care fund flows in many different ways. Federal, state, and local tax withholdings and health benefit contributions are removed from health care consumers' paychecks. Most health care consumers contribute to American health care ecosystem fund flows before they ever see a penny they've earned hit their bank account.

After earnings hit the bank accounts of American health care consumers, they continue to put money into the health care ecosystem whenever they utilize services. They do this primarily through co-payments, deductibles, and additional private spending on health care. The extra spending isn't included in the covered benefit package the American health care consumer has been paying into.

Covered benefits are likely selected from a small menu of options curated by employers. The menu of options is typically designed with no input from the consumer.

Once employers withhold consumers' earnings, they either retain it on their balance sheet to pay claims directly or transfer the funds to payers. Some withholdings from the consumers' paycheck collected by federal, state, and local authorities are also assigned to payers. Finally, several consumers also transfer funds directly to private payers to acquire additional benefit plans or expand coverage.

The federal government is one of the nation's largest employers and transfers funds to private payers. Those funds reflect the employer portion of the health benefit costs for acquiring health insurance and are separate from other federal government funds transfers to private payers.

Due to the current design of the Medicaid system, the federal government completes complex and opaque calculations to determine and ultimately transfer the federal "match" of funds to all states to administer Medicaid and related programs administered at the state level.

While the federal contribution to Medicaid is commonly referred to as a "match," in reality, the federal government finances the majority of all Medicaid spending. According to the Kaiser Family Foundation, in 2019, the federal government contributed anywhere from 52-percent of Medicaid spending, as was the case in Wyoming, to 78.9-percent of Medicaid spending, as was the case in New Mexico.

Those public and private payers accumulate funds and health care consumer lives. They proceed to establish thousands of different, primarily fee-for-service contracts with provider groups that offer the services in the various benefit packages they sold to the American health care consumers they represent.

Most of the contracts are complicated to construct and have nuanced variations based on many factors and conditions. Renegotiation of those contractual agreements typically occurs on an annual basis.

The nuanced variations and annual contracting cycles often cause both the payers and providers to increasingly pursue approaches to gaining negotiating leverage and a favorable outcome for their group. Standard techniques include hiring armies of esoteric knowledge experts—lawyers, consultants, financial professionals, health economists, former regulators, etcetera—and acquiring other American health care industry stakeholders to gain additional negotiating leverage.

Fee-for-service transaction complexity and the ensuing arms race to consolidate buying power to gain negotiating leverage continue to drive costs, prices, and spending higher while minimizing competition. These conditions enable the market failures that lead to the growth and continued success of the American health care cartel. A success that scales at the expense of consumers and taxpayers.

The inefficient and challenging evolution of the structure, design, and financing of the American health care ecosystem has led to significant complexity, rapid price growth, and persistent inequities. These issues are exacerbated when American health care collides with the hierarchy of White supremacy.

Since the providers with a treasure trove of data on American health care consumers know which consumers they can extract the most monetary value from, they exploit that information asymmetry whenever they can. They preferentially engage and serve American health care consumers they anticipate will provide more financial value at the point of service or when the provider entity seeks external monetary donations. While most providers aren't sophisticated enough to know precisely how much providing care to one patient will yield versus another patient, they use the source of insurance coverage and race as a proxy for which patients will likely deliver the greatest financial return.

Some providers often deliver higher quality service to consumers with private insurance and consumers who are White. American health care is primarily a commercial enterprise. And the American economy is capitalistic by design. As such, providers seek to attract more patients with private insurance that reimburse at rates that are more lucrative than the reimbursement rates public payers offer.

Since the wealth gap is so wide between White people and Black people, some providers seek to curry favor with more White people who they hope will donate funds to whatever "charitable" fundraising effort the providers have prioritized. Those fundraising efforts typically align with low-value capital projects like remodeled spaces named after the donors. The effects of this preferential treatment are reflected in the health outcomes achieved by members of the different groups. People with public insurance versus those with private insurance. White versus people of color, etcetera.

Providers that primarily work in the nursing home arena are the American health care cartel members that primarily discriminate between two different publicly funded health benefit plans and don't pay too much attention to private health benefit plans. Due to the various rules, benefit design, and reimbursement rates in the publicly funded Medicare and Medicaid programs, American health care cartel members that primarily operate in the nursing home arena preferentially deliver care to Medicare patients. They do this because they can extract the most economic rents from Medicare patients. Medicaid patients usually get the short end of every stick. Every single one. Exacerbating the crisis is the common practice of overtreatments and overbilling. Overtreatment occurs with

Medicare patients, while Medicaid patients in the same nursing home facilities are often ignored or offered skimpy services before their benefits run out. Medicaid patients literally get kicked to the curb or dumped in a shelter when their benefits run out. This scenario and the related malaise are enabled by the fee-for-service transaction system that reimburses certain activities while refusing payment for other activities. Lobbyists and other cartel members usually influence covered benefits.

American health care cartel members primarily focused on delivering services in the nursing home arena are particularly adept at maximizing revenues and profit per patient. The nursing home industry is also unique because most of the providers in the space operate as for-profit organizations. Their approach to classifying their organizations as for-profit entities is at least an authentic and self-aware take on their primary motivations and why they exist. This approach is a far cry from "non-profit" organizations in the provider space that operate in the same manner as for-profit organizations. Still, because of their "non-profit" status, they also get to run the donation "side hustle."

Not-for-profit hospitals have a sweet deal.

Unlike for-profit hospitals, not-for-profit hospitals pay no taxes.

They pay no state or federal income tax, no property tax, and no sales tax. They are supposed to reinvest in the surrounding community. They mostly reinvest in their gilded hospital-centric health system campuses.

Whether flying a for-profit or "non-profit" organization flag, American health care cartel members structure their organizations to operate in a manner that allows them to maximize revenues. Often, the approaches pursued to maximize revenues lead to good patient outcomes. In several instances, attempts to maximize revenues do not affect the patient's outcomes. With the worst encounters, attempts to maximize revenues result in horrible patient outcomes, including death.

The American health care ecosystem typically provides the best care to wealthy White males with commercial insurance and the worst levels of care to low-income Black females with no insurance. From access to treatments to demographic representation in clinical trials, wealthy White males receive significant favor from the American health care cartel. Low-income Black females are significantly disadvantaged by the American health care cartel.

The regulatory entities and technical systems that enable fee-for-service fund flows and transactions have gotten so complex that I can confidently state that there aren't any individuals or organizations capable of connecting all the dots. No one knows all the rules of engagement across the entire American health care ecosystem.

For example, almost every Federal agency and several state and local agencies have a role in enabling the functioning of fee-for-service fund flows and transactions in the American health care ecosystem. Collaboration and coordination among federal agencies is a complex feat to accomplish, even for simple objectives. We exacerbate the current crisis by attempting to layer the complexity of the federal bureaucracy on the complexity of fee-for-service fund flows and transactions. A calamity that results in ever-increasing prices, costs, and spending while consumer and taxpayer value erodes.

Due to the design of the incentive model and fee-for-service approaches to transactions, American health care cartel members profit when delivering curative care. They have more significant opportunities to capture economic rents when delivering expensive curative medicine to consumers that engage the American health care ecosystem. Chronically ill persons with certain comorbidities primarily consume

American health care cartel members' expensive curative medical services.

American health care consumers with chronic conditions and functional limitations usually make up more than 75-percent of the top 5-percent highest American health care consumers annually. Sadly, this sordid statistic persists as consumers in the groups mentioned above only represent about 10-percent of the rest of the population outside the top 5-percent of health care consumers every year.

Chronically ill health care consumers with functional limitations usually have unmet needs that go unaddressed by the medical delivery system financed by fee-for-service transactions. According to the Lewin Group, functional limitations are restrictions on physical activity (e.g., walking, bending, stooping), everyday life activity (e.g., work, housework, school), Activities of Daily Living (ADL), or Instrumental Activities of Daily Living (IADL). ADLs and IADLs are typically the class of activities essential to personal hygiene, grooming, and the process of entering into or getting out of bed.

There is typically no reimbursement for most activities impacted by functional limitations unless a patient is in a hospital setting. As such, providers have little incentive to provide services they won't collect reimbursement for when a patient isn't in a hospital setting.

Further, when a functionally limited person cannot obtain preventive care or experiences trauma (e.g., falls), they typically end up having to procure expensive curative treatments to address the trauma or poorly managed chronic illnesses. Under the fee-for-service system and the underlying contractual arrangements, service providers can extract significantly higher reimbursements for services rendered in increasingly acute medical services settings.

While providers swear an oath to "first do no harm," provider members of the American health care cartel are driven by capitalism and a desire to extract as much value as they are allowed to get away with from every encounter. Providers with incentives to operate in this manner are also partially driven by a base sense of self-preservation.

Long Term Care (LTC) facilities are the provider cohort notorious for typically exploiting the plight of the functionally limited population. Often presenting themselves as homely and pleasant, nursing homes, assisted living facilities, and other institutions of that ilk increasingly extract economic rents while harm comes to those in their care. Making matters worse is the level of abuse and neglect that sometimes occurs in those environments. Abuse and neglect are personified in the high mortality rate of nursing home residents infected with COVID-19.

While most functionally limited and elderly persons would prefer to stay in their homes and receive home-based care, the American health care cartel can extract greater economic rents when health care consumers are institutionalized. As such, the American health care cartel typically resists innovation that would disrupt the status quo while consumers and taxpayers continue to suffer the consequences.

Unfortunately, many providers who choose not to play by the American health care cartel rules are likely to succumb to financial pressures or lose comparative advantage in their respective markets. Exacerbating this calamity are scenarios where providers cannot keep up with the additional investments their competitors can make due to the financial windfall associated with the American health care cartel's approach to doing business. As such, providers who aren't part of the American health care cartel eventually go out of business or sell out to a dominant provider in the American health care cartel. Additional suitors in the mix to acquire such providers are other American health care cartel members who have a myriad of reasons for wanting a seat in the provider section of the American health care cartel table.

Unfortunately for health care consumers and taxpayers, despite the significant health spending enabled by members of the American health care cartel, the American health care ecosystem continues to deliver suboptimal results. Estimates indicate that access to medical services accounts for only 10-percent of what keeps people healthy. Meanwhile, almost 90-percent of health spending is focused on the delivery of medical services and institutional care.

This calamity worsens because the healthy behaviors that account for 50-percent of what leads to good health outcomes are only typically accessible to certain members of American society. Accessibility is primarily determined by where those American community members fall on the societal hierarchy propagated by White supremacy.

For example, it is more likely that the average White person can engage in healthy behaviors like exercising, eating nutritious food, and advancing their life skills. Unfortunately for most Black people, American institutions and organizations that promote White supremacy disadvantage Black people from engaging in similar healthy behaviors.

The average Black person lacks safe spaces to exercise outdoors and has limited access to indoor exercise equipment. Either due to neighborhood violence (e.g., gangs and White vigilantes with guns) or the risk of interactions with police that could prove fatal, some Black people are apprehensive about being outdoors. Many Black people lack financial resources to cover expenses associated with living in city dwellings or suburban communities with indoor gyms.

When Black people can afford to live in city dwellings or suburban communities with indoor gyms, they often have to deal with racial microaggressions. Often contending with confrontations with other patrons demanding they prove they are authorized to be there. In different scenarios, non-Black patrons of the indoor gyms choose to leave once a Black person arrives. Classic manifestations of common microaggressions Black people face in public spaces.

In addition to challenges many Black people face avoiding sedentary lifestyles, most predominantly Black communities are nutritious food deserts. This unfortunate reality leaves Black people living in those communities surrounded mainly by unhealthy food options. Overall, too many Americans are nutritious food insecure because, besides being surrounded by unhealthy food options, many lack the work-life balance to prepare healthy, home-cooked meals.

Finally, American institutions that promote White supremacy continue to undermine the health and well-being of Black people by routinely limiting the opportunities Black people have to advance their life skills or maximize their full potential.

Compared to other "first world" nations in the Organization of Economic Cooperation and Development (OECD), America consistently ranks lower than almost all its peers in all health outcomes categories. The only category where America consistently ranks higher than other OECD nations is in per capita expenditure on health care and the percentage of Gross Domestic Product (GDP) allocated to national health care spending.

America's performance and rankings continue to decline for life expectancy at birth, Infant mortality, obesity rates, and proportion of the populace afflicted with multiple chronic conditions. The American health care cartel ensures that more spending shifts to the bloated and misguided

American health care ecosystem that continues to deliver bad outcomes for American consumers and taxpayers.

Further exacerbating the crisis is the American health care cartel's desire to ensure more spending shifts to the delivery of medical services. The American health care industry continues to underperform its peers in the OECD that spend considerably less on delivering medical services. Compared to other OECD countries, America is typically either ranked in the middle of the pack or close to dead last for quality of care, access, efficiency, equity, and healthy lives.

Worsening these suboptimal outcomes are the persistently higher prices paid in America. Higher prices contribute to low-value spending estimated to represent about 30-percent of annual health care spending in America. The disparities seen between prices in America and other OECD countries indicate that "competition" between providers in America has failed to control consumer prices like it has for different business sectors in the American economy. When compared to citizens of OECD countries, American consumers routinely pay higher prices for precisely the same unit of care. A reality enabled by the stranglehold the American health care cartel has on the American health care industry.

Despite the high prices, elevated spending, and the bloated size of the American health care ecosystem, American consumers are getting less for their health spending. At the same time, essential services remain underfunded because health care and related expenditures continue to take a larger share of American GDP, federal, state, and local budgets.

Over the last couple of decades, hospitals, physicians and clinics, and prescription drugs have seen exponential growth in spending across all three categories. Health care spending on hospital services typically represents about 30-percent of national health care spending, while money spent on physicians and clinics typically represents 20-percent.

Macro calculations of money spent on prescription drugs are typically around 10-percent of overall health care spending. However, the channel economics of the pharmaceutical industry makes it challenging to ascertain what proportion of the health care spending on hospitals, physicians, or clinics is a derivative of drugs—pharmaceuticals, therapeutics, etcetera.

Exacerbating the malaise is the unfortunate reality that more than 25-percent of the federal budget funds the bloated American health care ecosystem. In addition to the 25-percent allocation to health care spending, more than 50-percent of the rest of the federal budget goes to poorly designed and unsustainable entitlement programs and bloated military spending. The military-industrial complex bolsters military spending.

Congress directs the majority of the federal budget to bloated, poorly designed American institutions that propagate the hierarchy of White supremacy. As such, America barely invests more than 10-percent of the federal budget into assets and resources capable of preparing the American economy to prosper as the world transitions to the next industrial revolution.

After the big three spending categories—entitlements, health care, military—are sated, interest payment on America's debt is the fourth largest federal spending category. As America's debt continues to balloon and deficits persist, I assume the forces that retain a stranglehold on federal spending will continue to eke out savings from other categories of federal spending while mostly ignoring the unsustainable growth of the big four.

These mediocre outcomes are by design. The health care, military, and entitlements industrial complexes are preoccupied with growing their share of the pie regardless of the devastating impact their greed has on American prosperity, quality of life, or future outlook. America's outstanding debt liabilities and related interest payments are a negative externality of a federal spending ecosystem beholden to special interests and the advancement of institutions designed to serve the hierarchy of White supremacy. Redesigning those institutions to address challenges faced by all Americans will be better for the nation and the world.

Another driver of the delivery of expensive curative medicine is mental disorders in chronically ill persons. Diagnosed or otherwise. It is materially more challenging for people struggling with mental illnesses to adhere to evidence-based treatment or prevention care paths. While America continues to experience a behavioral and mental health crisis, it has underinvested in its mental health infrastructure over the years. While there are many reasons for the underinvestment, the fee-for-service fund flows, legacy technology systems, and regulatory framework are the main culprits. Regulations and legacy technology systems weren't designed or integrated with mental health infrastructure over time.

Extracting more revenue from the health care ecosystem is easier when delivering medical services to address issues ailing the physical body. As such, American health care cartel members saw little value in advancing mental health care infrastructure as they orchestrated the evolution of the cash cow known as the physical health care delivery ecosystem.

Exacerbating this calamity is the incentive model that enables American health care cartel members to harvest more money by addressing physical trauma suffered by health care consumers with untreated mental disorders than attempting to diagnose or treat the mental illness. As such, cartel members doubled down on investments and approaches to boost their financial position and continue to resist efforts to integrate physical and psychological health care ecosystems. One of the primary reasons the physical and mental health care ecosystem wasn't integrated and remains disconnected is because the current design empowers American health care cartel members to extract greater economic rents.

Even after the Affordable Care Act (ACA) was signed into law and renewed focus placed on integrating physical and mental health ecosystems, a material deficit remains. We are yet to actualize the infrastructure required to make meaningful integration a reality. At this juncture, I'm not even sure American health care cartel members can successfully integrate the physical and mental health care ecosystems even if they had the incentive to do so.

One of the main drivers of the lack of infrastructure is the extreme shortage of clinical and general mental health professionals. Exacerbating the need is the high rate of clinician burnout and rising rates of suicide death among physicians, especially physicians who primarily support the mental health care ecosystem.

According to the 2021 Medscape National Physician Burnout and Suicide Report, 41-percent of the psychiatrists surveyed indicated they felt burned out.

One psychiatrist shared that they were "tired and discouraged," expressing the stress the burnout places on their marriage while sharing how hard it was to get out of bed to go to work.

A more sobering statistic from the same report was that 15-percent of the psychiatrists surveyed indicated that they had entertained thoughts of suicide.

According to the CDC, suicide is the second most common cause of death for 10-to 34-year-olds in America.

The medical training model embraced by the American health care cartel is designed to reduce the quality of life of trainees.

A model designed to increase mental stress.

A model designed to increase indebtedness.

A model designed to preserve the status quo.

The timing of the most rigorous training a physician endures typically occurs between the ages of 23 and 34. Physicians who train in America are among the cohort of Americans who decide to commit suicide between 10 and 34.

Suicidality is pervasive across the different stages of medical training.

From medical school to Residency and beyond, physicians often have to contend with environmental factors that increase their risk of committing suicide.

"As things are now, no one can tell who members of Congress are responsible to, except that it does not often appear to be to the people. Everyone else is represented in Washington by a rich and powerful lobby, it seems. But there is no lobby for the people." – Rep. Shirley Chisholm

Physician Burnout

"The value of a college education (or any education) is not the learning of many facts, but the training of the mind to think." – Albert Einstein

Demand for physicians continues to grow faster than supply. As such, a shortfall of thousands of physicians exists in several health care markets across America. These shortfalls are getting worse over time. These shortfalls exist by design. These shortfalls exist because the American health care cartel profits from the existence of the shortfall.

Physician shortfalls are most prevalent in underserved communities of color and rural areas. The persistence of physician shortfalls results in millions of health care consumers not receiving adequate or equitable access to preventive health care and services.

According to the American Association of Medical Colleges (AAMC), America will have to contend with a projected physician shortage of between 54,100 and 139,000 physicians by 2033. The shifting demographics of American society are exacerbating this crisis. As the American population ages, national birth rates are dropping. The worsening caregiver shortage worsens the adverse impacts of physician shortfalls in health care markets across America. Current trends are troubling.

In addition to the shifting demographics, other factors negatively impact the physician demand-supply imbalance in America. Structural processes that propagate White supremacy, policies that artificially restrict physician supply, and physician burnout are some of the primary reasons why the physician demand-supply imbalance persists in several health care markets in America.

The structural processes designed into the American professional medical journey propagate White supremacy and enables policies that artificially restrict physician supply. Racial disparities in the physician workforce and training pipeline also exacerbate this problem.

Racial disparities in physician training and career outcomes are a troubling manifestation of cancer metastasizing at the intersection of White supremacy and American health care.

According to a 2018 report published by AAMC, Black physicians accounted for 5-percent of the 918,547 active physicians in the American health care ecosystem. Meanwhile, White physicians represent 56-percent of all active physicians.

The physician pipeline isn't much better. Of the 22,239 students enrolled into medical schools in the 2020/2021 academic year, AAMC reported that 8-Percent identified as Black and 45-percent identified as White. Black and White students are proportionally under-represented. Asians who account for 22-percent of those who enroll in medical school are over-represented.

I wasn't able to find research reports that highlighted the rates at which Black medical school graduates Match to Residency programs. I assume the proportional representation of Black first-year residents is worse than Black students' rates that enrolled into American medical schools.

If the numbers were commendable, I assume The National Resident Matching Program® (NRMP®), also known as The Match®, would proudly promote those numbers on its website and published reports. Maybe I just didn't look hard enough.

I posit that although less than 50-percent of the students who enroll in medical school identify as White, implicit biases and the American health care cartel tip the scales during the Resident Matching process. Thus, more than 50-percent of all Residency spot awardees are usually White medical school graduates. As the doctrine of White supremacy dictates, White people, particularly White males, are advantaged throughout the Resident Matching process. Black people, especially Black males, are disadvantaged throughout the Resident Matching process.

The racial disparities achieved by the Resident Matching process, including its underlying Nobel Prize-winning algorithm, are designed to achieve the outcomes mentioned above.

Coded bias?

Joy Buolamwini and The Algorithmic Justice League should investigate.

The Resident Matching process is the lever that elitist White supremacists and the American health care cartel use to control physicians' supply and racial diversity across the American health care ecosystem. Racial and gender disparities in the Resident Matching process are among the most corrosive manifestations of cancer metastasizing at the intersection of White supremacy and American health care.

Supply and demand economics dictate that all else being equal; prices rise when supply is constrained, and demand increases. The mission of the American health care cartel is to raise prices and spending on "health care." That's why the American health care cartel supports the current design of the Resident Matching process and the American Professional Medical Training (PMT) journey.

The hierarchy of the practice of medicine puts physicians, especially specialists, at the top of the totem pole and as leaders of the clinical care team. Consequently, physicians are a revered profession. A profession the wealthiest and Whitest members of American society are best positioned to pursue. But for their mediocrity, low resilience, and a plethora of options, I assume more elitist White supremacists would have embarked on an American PMT journey. To propagate White supremacy, elitist White supremacists endorse the current design of the Resident Matching process and the American PMT journey.

Most medical school faculty positions remain overwhelmingly White and male. Like most professional journeys where entry and career progression are determined by "kingmakers" already in the profession, implicit biases, especially similar-to-me bias, have an overwhelming effect on who gets to enter and who gets to succeed. And on decision-making more broadly.

Similar-to-me bias manifests when people disproportionately favor individuals who are like them.

In the American professional medical journey, similar-to-me bias is pervasive and reflected in the racial composition of medical school students and graduates who are advantaged to enroll and trainees advantaged to Match to Residency programs. Beyond racial disparities in entry and progression, like most White and male-dominated professions, gender bias is similarly pervasive.

The American Professional Medical Training (PMT) design is convoluted, lengthy, and expensive. Most Black people and females are disadvantaged from starting the process or successfully advancing through it.

The widening wealth gap between White people and Black people in America is one of the most pervasive, sinister, and consequential manifestations of White supremacy.

Most Black people can't afford to start or complete the American PMT process. Many that embark on the American professional medical journey soon acquire copious amounts of debt. Those copious amounts of debt often turn to permanent financial ruin for those who don't complete the American PMT process or advance into the financially rewarding portion of the American professional medical journey.

As a result of centuries of oppression, exploitation, and theft, Black people worldwide are disproportionately low-income and impoverished.

While many seek alternative facts and concoct theories to justify racial disparities' pervasiveness in wealth and life outcomes, the root cause is the propagation of White supremacy. Alternative facts and theories are merely symptoms and manifestations of White supremacy.

Many lack the internal fortitude or depth of critical thought to acknowledge this truth. Those people swiftly embrace alternative facts and theories conjured by institutions who seek to shift the blame elsewhere.

Others are shameless capitalists who lack the wisdom to pursue other "hustles." Many who exploit this shameful hustle only have the intellectual capacity to succeed in careers where the "critical skill" is one's ability to articulate an opinion. An opinion that doesn't have to be rooted in truth. Viewpoints that don't even have to be factually accurate.

For alternate root causes to be assumed to credible, one must embrace delusional theories propagated by the institution of White supremacy. Delusional theories abound. For example, some believe that Black people are inherently anti-intellectual underachievers. They think Black people love embracing and exploiting the "trappings of poverty." The cause of all this? High melanin ratios and Black culture. Foolishness.

The ratio of melanin in a person's skin isn't inherently predictive or indicative of socioeconomic outcomes.

The prevalence of White supremacy is.

<u>The recent global history of European imperialism and colonialism is.</u>

People preoccupied with symptoms while ignoring or dismissing root causes are misguided at best and treacherous in worst-case scenarios. "Dudes" and "dudettes" have a rudimentary understanding of White supremacy and are Ill-equipped to recognize all the negative externalities derived from White supremacy.

I posit that the deluded approach to reasoning embodied in White supremacist logic is pervasive across the mindset of all "dudes" and "dudettes" because they are prone to believe other antiquated constructs and hierarchies propagated by society. Constructs and hierarchies like misogyny, bigotry, and patriarchy.

American government policy exacerbates wealth disparities enabled by the myriad of industrial complexes that control American institutions. The design of those American institutions by industrial complexes allows them to shower White people with taxpayer dollars. At the same time, they refuse to allocate taxpayer dollars to benefit people of color meaningfully.

Government and community spending on the law enforcement industrial complex has one of the lowest socioeconomic multiplier effects on American society. However, any nation designed to propagate primal White supremacy™ continues to overinvest in its law enforcement infrastructure. Doing so ensures that mediocre White "dudes" and "dudettes" have a steady income source and are in positions of authority.

Mediocre White "dudes" or "dudettes" are in positions of authority throughout the law enforcement industrial complex. From the officer in the juvenile correction facility to the justice appointed to the U.S. Supreme Court, the primary "skill" it takes to "excel" in law enforcement is the ability to assess situations, issue commands, and enforce the law.

Assessing situations is inherent to any rational human and essential to navigating human interactions. Issuing commands and enforcing the law aren't inherently valuable skills.

Appropriately designed laws, institutions, and incentives eliminate the need for significant human involvement to encourage people to comply with the law.

The land of the "free" incarcerates more of its citizens than any other nation on earth.

The land of the "free" <u>imprisons more than 25-percent of the world's prisoners</u>.

Overinvesting human capital in professions centered on issuing commands and enforcing the law merely to propagate White supremacy often produces unfortunate outcomes and devastating consequences.

Unfortunate outcomes manifest as White "dudes" and "dudettes" trapped in a vocation or career that doesn't maximize their potential. White "dudes" and "dudettes" aren't challenged to be their most valuable selves while deteriorating in the law enforcement industrial complex. They can be valuable contributors to American society, but their true potential remains hidden from American society. The doctrine of White supremacy strikes again.

America would be a more prosperous nation if it decided to maximize the potential of its population of mediocre White "dudes" and "dudettes." Instead, it condemns them to low-value contributions manifested as servitude to the law enforcement industrial complex.

Devastating consequences manifest as Black and Brown masses trapped by a law enforcement industrial complex that oppresses, exploits, and dehumanizes America's Black and Brown people.

Black and Brown masses are trapped so that mediocre White "dudes" and "dudettes" are gainfully employed. As the scheme scales, the law enforcement industrial complex captures a larger share of federal, state, and local budgets.

White people proportionally and in absolute terms consume more illicit and harmful drugs—including drugs that should be illicit but are "legal" since White people like them—than any other racial group in America. The design of the law enforcement industrial complex enables it to propagate White supremacy. As such, White people aren't the largest racial group prosecuted or incarcerated for drug-related offenses.

America would be a more prosperous nation if it sought to maximize the potential of its Black and Brown masses. Instead, it condemns them to low-value contributions embodied in their implicit role as fodder. As fodder, they are the readily available material used to supply the heavy demand that justifies the existence of the law enforcement industrial complex. As the scheme scales, capital allocation increases.

Social engineering designed to uphold White supremacy by empowering mediocre White "dudes" and "dudettes" does little to prosper America. And now that the world is transitioning to the next industrial revolution, elevating mediocrity is much more detrimental.

Power accrues to the wealthy in a capitalistic society.

The wealthy have significant privilege.

The wealthy weaponize their wealth to disadvantage the underprivileged masses.

Social conditioning trains the underprivileged masses to ignore viable paths to overcoming their oppressors while fixating on pointless dialogue and building bridges to nowhere.

The last several paragraphs might appear out of place. They aren't. I'm putting forward the argument that Black people are disadvantaged from accumulating wealth and avoiding criminalization in American society. The wealth and clean criminal record are required to complete the American PMT process.

Black people are set up to fail their attempts to complete the American PMT process. The dwindling representation of Black people in the medical profession is a symptom of that devastating reality.

A devastating reality that significantly impacts Black people's care when they engage the American health care ecosystem. Dwindling representation also affects the efficacy of medical interventions developed and promoted, cures pursued, treatment protocols rendered, and disorders researched etcetera.

Beyond delays in adherence to evidence-based clinical guidelines, people of color and females of all races are also disadvantaged because the evidence informing the guideline isn't typically representative. Widely accepted "evidence-based" clinical guidelines aren't usually representative of all the populations those "evidence-based" clinical guidelines are supposed to serve.

Many Americans are yet to evolve to empathize with people they can't quickly identify with or relate to in any context.

A medical and scientific community that is predominantly White and male is ill-equipped to adequately serve an American population that is increasingly female and imbued with higher ratios of melanin.

That's the truth.

The whole truth.

Nothing but the truth.

Physician burnout manifests for many reasons. Similar to the American professional sports journey athletes embark on, physicians endure a grueling American professional medical journey with many inflection points that can prematurely terminate their journey. Many journeys end arbitrarily, sometimes due to no fault of the physician or athlete. The "powers that be" may decide the physician or athlete "isn't a fit" or "made of the right stuff." Dashing their hopes, dreams, and preferred professional identity with a single, critical rejection letter.

The Residency Matching process is very similar to the National Football League (NFL) draft. Physicians and athletes both interview with several potential organizations looking to fill a couple of spots. Most of the evaluators in both institutions are overwhelmingly White and male. Although physicians and athletes express their preference and rank organizations they would like to work for, the power to choose largely rests with the selecting organization and not the physician or athlete. Upon selection, the physician or athlete moves to the city or state where their employer is based.

The path to gainful employment as a physician or NFL player is strikingly similar. Those who dedicate their lives to achieving gainful employment as a physician or NFL player face a crisis of confidence and languish when the "powers that be" decide not to let them into the fold.

While there are many similarities, athletes have some rights to appeal draft day decisions and are richly rewarded after being drafted. Physicians have no rights of appeal and aren't richly rewarded after Matching to a Residency program. Greater financial rewards are available after Residency is completed unless additional training is required after Residency.

Residency rewards physicians with more grueling training, the opportunity to earn minimum wage per hour worked, a full embrace of depressingly low quality-of-life, and a continuation of the misery-inducing work-life balance designed into most Residency programs.

My family and I had first-hand exposure to the malaise of the current design of the American PMT process. Thankfully we were more fortunate than most. Pretty much everything worked out as planned. I shudder to think about what might have happened to our family if any of those inflection points didn't turn out in our favor after all the hard work Bolanle put in and the sacrifices our family made.

Though grateful, our family remains severely challenged by our experience with the American PMT process. Adding strain to my relationship with Bolanle were the 36-hour shifts, board examination prep, obstacles, and nerve-racking inflection points designed into the American PMT process.

With hard work, perseverance, faith in God, and the support of our families, after graduating with her bachelor's degree from Howard University, Bolanle completed 4-years of medical school and graduated second in her class. She won many awards throughout medical school and graduated with zero debt. The awards and scholarships she earned in medical school were sufficient to cover most of her tuition and fees. Her parents took care of the rest.

She Matched to her preferred Residency program.

She completed 3-years of Internal Medicine (IM) Residency.

She became the first Black female Chief Resident in the history of the program.

While it's a great honor to be the first Black insert title here, it remains a signal of how much farther Black people still have to go to close the achievement gap in America.

After her year as Chief Resident, she successfully Matched to her preferred Cardiology Fellowship program. Cardiology Fellowship programs are highly coveted 3-to-4-year ordeals that very few women are ever empowered to pursue. It's not that they aren't capable; instead, the prevalence of many factors primarily caused by gender biases in the evaluation and selection process is why most women don't Match to Cardiology Fellowship programs.

As she concludes the final year of her 12-year American PMT process, I am immensely proud of her and her accomplishments. She isn't just a medical professional; she is also a wife to me, a mother to our three beautiful daughters, and a daughter to our parents.

Completing her journey required a lot of hard work, sacrifice, perseverance, and favor.

Favor from God and humans.

I'm eternally grateful that the many inflection points along the way weren't too disruptive to our family plans. Family and life planning that too many trainees have to sacrifice or put on hold to successfully complete the American PMT process.

A family and life plan many may never actualize as a result.

Burnout starts during medical school.

It calcifies during Residency.

Subsequently, burnout becomes debilitating during the years of training and medical practice that occur after Residency. There are many reasons why physician burnout is pervasive in American health care and often drives physicians to the brink.

The design of the American PMT process.

The obscene financial burden associated with the American PMT process.

Trauma from overexposure to human suffering.

The peculiarities associated with the practice of medicine in America.

All these factors often drive many physicians to the brink. The American health care cartel predominantly saddles those who complete the American PMT process with stress, fatigue, and copious amounts of debt. Physicians consumed by stress, fatigue, and indebtedness aren't inclined to pursue initiatives to disrupt the status quo.

Some physicians revel in their traumatic experiences going through the American PMT process like a badge of honor. The American PMT process conditions many to be risk-averse. By the time they cross the finish line of the PMT process, they are ready to finally pursue the family and life plans they put on hold for so long. The PMT process can be so toxic that some physicians complete the process filled with disdain and regret.

One of our family friends, a general surgeon, candidly shared that she wouldn't sacrifice her firstborn son at the altar of the American PMT process. She is not alone. Several surveys indicate that physicians are increasingly suggesting that they wouldn't encourage people they care about to pursue medicine. Others are stating that they would choose an alternate career path if they had the chance to remake their career path.

A review of recent statistics reveals another sobering reality. According to Medscape's 2020 National Physicians Burnout and Depression Report, of all the physicians surveyed, 42-percent reported that they felt burned out.

Those rates of burnout vary by gender and generation. According to the survey, women (48-percent) were more likely to report feelings of burnout than men (37-percent). Physicians from Generation X (48-percent) were the most likely to report feelings of burnout, followed by baby boomers (39-percent) and millennials (38-percent).

Worse yet, physicians are committing suicide at alarming rates.

According to the American Hospital Association (AHA), approximately 400 physicians die by suicide each year, while hundreds more harbor severe thoughts of suicide.

The suicide completion rate among doctors is 44% higher than the expected population. Female physicians have a higher suicide completion rate than male physicians. The AHA report indicated that stress, burnout, and trauma all contribute to the aforementioned sobering statistics.

Experts expect that the traumatic events many physicians and clinical care teams experienced during the COVID-19 pandemic would likely worsen those sobering statistics.

"It is not necessary to change. Survival is not mandatory."
– W. Edwards Deming

Roles and Incentives of Key Stakeholders

"There are no saints in the American health care ecosystem. We are all sinners. Different stakeholders are simply focused on increasing the influence of their group and related economic rents."

It is widely known that consumer spending accounts for more than two-thirds of the U.S. economy. As such, the growth of the U.S. economy is reliant on the American consumer's ability to consume goods and services. Instead of shifting towards more balance and a production-centric economy, America continues to double down on consumer spending as its engine for economic growth.

Focusing the American economy on consumer spending is a reckless decision because America remains burdened by trade and budget deficits as well as trillions of dollars in mounting debt. A debt burden exacerbated by the trillions of dollars in economic stimulus injected into the U.S. economy as financial markets cratered at the onset of the COVID-19 pandemic in America. Although we are a year removed from the initial round of economic stimulus, it is unclear how much more stimulus will be applied to give the largest economy in the world another "shot in the arm."

While debt-financed spending isn't inherently harmful, especially in low-interest-rate environments, America's national debt was incurred because decision-makers primarily enacted policies designed to enrich the wealthiest individuals and corporations in America. Exacerbating the ongoing crisis is that a non-trivial portion of America's debt-financed spending was incurred to support consumer spending. Consumption of goods and services primarily produced in other countries. A pattern of behavior that results in America incurring trillions of dollars in debt, underinvesting in its infrastructure, and essentially paying for infrastructure development in production-centric economies like China.

Consumption of health care goods and services currently accounts for almost 20-percent of American Gross Domestic Product (GDP). It continues to rise. The American health care ecosystem's incentive models and fund flows encourage higher volumes of goods and services to be delivered regardless of need.

Absent any intervention, the unsustainable growth of the American health care ecosystem will become the leading contributor to the acceleration of the demise of American prosperity.

American society bears its health care costs. This reality contributes to America's lack of comparative advantage in the domestic production of goods and services. Those health care costs are often included in labor costs. They are also a direct expense that burdens all organizations operating in America.

As America's path to prosperity remains on life support, the American health care cartel continues to laugh all the way to the bank.

As America perfects its self-defeating act, production-centric economies (especially the ones that create many of the goods Americans consume) wonder if America will ever figure out how to win this game in the long run.

Key members of the American health care industry aren't organized or financed to deliver higher-value care. Especially the type that reduces unnecessary medical service utilization and costs. Excessive medical service utilization and expenses account for the lion's share of the waste in the American health care ecosystem.

In addition to the American health care ecosystem stakeholders represented in the American health care cartel, the essential stakeholder often intentionally excluded from the decision-making table is the patient.

Patients primarily come from the ranks of the American health care consumer. Some fly into America from other countries. But for the demand created by patients, most American health care cartel members in the payer, provider, and producer categories would have little reason to exist.

In most instances, the patient is on the menu. At the same time, the American health care cartel devises increasingly opaque ways to exploit the appetizer, entrée, and dessert they choose to dine on through multiple courses of health reform flings, protracted relationships, and bitter divorces.

The American spirit is entrepreneurial by nature, so it breaks my heart to think about the millions of Americans trapped in thankless jobs simply because they can't afford to take the financial risk associated with pursuing entrepreneurship. Worsening the financial risk are devastating outcomes associated with engaging the American health care ecosystem as an uninsured or underinsured person.

Even with "adequate" insurance, some medical expenses and debt continue to eviscerate patient budgets and savings, often resulting in bankruptcies. The complexity, high prices, and inequities associated with the functioning of the American health care ecosystem exist and persist for many reasons.

One of the driving forces behind the pervasiveness of the complexity, high prices, and inequities are the roles and incentives of key stakeholders in the American health care ecosystem.

Key stakeholders are the architects of the way the American health care ecosystem currently functions. While all key stakeholders have potent levers to pull in efforts to advantage their stakeholder group, some key stakeholders are more adept at pulling those levers than others.

Profiles of key stakeholders in the American health care ecosystem.

1. **Patients.** (consumers)
   a. <u>Mostly cares about</u>: Access to reliable, convenient, and affordable health care. Wants to pay less while getting more for their money.
   b. <u>Evidence for action</u>: Trusts physicians and clinical teams, their community of family and friends, and propaganda from mass media outlets for insights on what works.
   c. <u>Primary motivation</u>: Pursuing improved health outcomes, well-being, and better quality of life conveniently and affordably.
   d. <u>Challenges</u>: Minimal market power. Limited agency to pursue consumer-centric care. Complicated access to personalized information on higher-value care paths. The focus of significant and exploitative marketing efforts designed to enable a desire to consume lower-value health products and services.

2. **Purchasers.** (employers, government)
   a. <u>Mostly cares about</u>: Reducing health care benefit spending.
   b. <u>Evidence for action</u>: Viable business case for cost-savings by any means, inclusive of cost-shifting to beneficiaries and covert quid pro quo agreements with other stakeholders.
   c. <u>Primary motivation</u>: Providing attractive benefit options to employees and reducing the impact of health benefits on profit growth and financial sustainability.
   d. <u>Challenges</u>: Minimal expertise in benefit design. Limited leverage in negotiations and contracting with third-party health benefits administrators. Structural barriers to extracting greater value from payers.
   Note: *Some self-insured employers negotiate directly with providers and producers.*

3. **Payers.** (insurers, public or private insurance agencies)
   a. <u>Mostly cares about</u>: Developing tools, resources, and market power to improve negotiating leverage with providers and producers. Extracting higher payments from purchasers. Lowering payouts to patients, providers, and producers.
   b. <u>Evidence for action</u>: Viable business case for commanding lower reimbursement for products and services from providers and producers.
   c. <u>Primary motivation</u>: Paying less in claims than received in premium payments.
   d. <u>Challenges</u>: Susceptible to market pressures and changing regulations. Some stakeholders desire to transition from fee-for-service transactions and incentives.
4. **Providers.** (health systems, nursing homes, clinical care teams, etcetera)
   a. <u>Mostly cares about</u>: Developing tools, resources, and market power to improve negotiating leverage with payers, purchasers, and producers.
   b. <u>Evidence for action</u>: Viable business case for commanding higher reimbursement for services. Patterns of behavior that lead to revenue and profit margin growth achieved by peers and competitors.
   c. <u>Primary motivation</u>: Sustaining revenues and profit margins by mainly delivering curative clinical services and improving health care outcomes.
   d. <u>Challenges</u>: Susceptible to market pressures and changing regulations. Reimbursement complexity.
5. **Producers.** (medical supply, pharmaceuticals, information technology, etcetera)
   a. <u>Mostly cares about</u>: Developing products and delivering services and convincing patients, purchases, payers, and providers to increase utilization and payments for the products and services offered.

b. <u>Evidence for action</u>: Viable business case to justify R&D and marketing spend that will likely be passed on to consumers.
c. <u>Primary motivation</u>: Increasing market share, revenue, and profits.
d. <u>Challenges</u>: Susceptible to market pressures and a changing regulatory environment of payment and clinical delivery reform.

While many American health care ecosystem stakeholders and interlopers fall outside the five highlighted groups, I wouldn't consider those interlopers as being essential to determining the outcome of American health reform efforts. On the other hand, key stakeholders play a substantial role in determining how the American health care ecosystem is designed and functions.

Unfortunately, key stakeholders are conditioned and incentivized to follow specific behavior patterns. Behavior patterns rooted in leaders of key stakeholder groups' decisions to remain complicit in propagating White supremacy across American society.

Except for people who cannot work, patients primarily choose who their purchaser representatives are by the employer they decide to work for and the state they choose to reside. American patients also have the power to select who their purchaser representatives are in the government.

American patients primarily exercise this right in local, state, and national elections. Elected officials voted into office by American patients appoint and hire other public servants to support their efforts. Public servants have significant influence over the hiring of senior members of the civil service.

Senior members of the civil service approve the hiring of less senior civil servants and oversee the work of the entire government workforce.

Public and civil servants are responsible for implementing the policy and regulatory priorities of the elected officials put in positions of power and authority.

Those public and civil servants control the design and functioning of the American health care ecosystem.

Unfortunately for patients and American health care consumers, many elected officials have louder voices ringing in their ears. Unfortunately, those Louder voices are competing with the voices of American patients and consumers crying out for help. Louder voices drowning out the voices of American patients who:

Stood in line.

Volunteered their time.

Donated to campaigns.

Those louder voices drown out the voices of American patients who cast the ballots that put the elected officials in office. Campaign finance corruption, partisan gerrymandering, and voter suppression laws are the pre-existing condition causing those louder voices to drown out the cries of patients and American health care consumers.

Those pre-existing conditions are rooted in America's misguided infatuation with upholding White supremacy.

A pre-existing condition that is preventing the nation from establishing an equitable, merit-based, American democracy.

American health care costs are borne by society.

This reality creates a free-rider problem.

Patients are incentivized to maximize their consumption of health care services while seeking to minimize their direct out-of-pocket spending on health care services.

All American health care ecosystem stakeholders act as incentivized. Patients too.

Patient consumption patterns typically correlate with direct out-of-pocket liability to the patient. Providers and producers are aware of this reality. They routinely implement wide-ranging strategies to minimize patients' direct out-of-pocket expenses while maximizing economic rents extracted from purchasers and payers.

Most patients have different medical service consumption patterns before they hit their annual out-of-pocket maximum versus after meeting their yearly deductibles and other out-of-pocket expenditures.

An October 2020 Issue Brief published by EBRI examined the extent to which members who satisfy their plan deductible continue to discriminate when it comes to services used. EBRI is a nonpartisan, tax-exempt organization created in 1978 to contribute to sound employee benefit programs and public policy through independent, objective, fact-based research and education.

The study compared the use of six commonly over-utilized imaging, screening, and pre-surgery testing services among 1.5 million individuals enrolled in commercial health plans. One group of study participants had satisfied their deductible, and the other group had not. EBRI reported that the likelihood of receiving low-value health care services increased by as much as 83 percent, depending on the service, for those who had satisfied their plan's deductible relative to those who had not.

The two primary purchasers in the American health care ecosystem are employers and the government.

According to recent Kaiser Family Foundation (KFF) data, more than 156 million people in America receive employer-sponsored health benefits. Employers usually work through intermediaries to source and select the health benefit plans they offer their employees. Other employers form group purchasing alliances to increase their negotiating leverage. Some larger employers choose to self-insure and self-administer the benefit programs they provide to their employees. While neither approach innately offers advantages to their employees, self-insured employers have a little more control over what they include in covered health benefits for their employees.

Excluding the uninsured population, about a third of all Americans utilize government-furnished health care benefits. And federal health spending accounts for almost a third of national health spending.

To address coverage gaps or retain additional flexibility, patients often combine their government-furnished health benefits with employer-sponsored health benefits.

<u>Major government health programs</u>.

Medicare. Created to serve senior citizens.

Medicaid. Created to serve the most vulnerable people in society.

State Children's Health Insurance Program (SCHIP). Created to support vulnerable children.

Department of Defense TRICARE and TRICARE for Life programs (DOD TRICARE). Created to support active-duty military families and retirees.

Veterans Health Administration (VHA). Created to serve vulnerable and service-disabled veterans.

Indian Health Service (IHS). Created to serve vulnerable Native American communities.

Federal Bureau of Prisons (BOP). Created to serve people incarcerated in federal prisons.

Different federal agencies run these government health programs.

Federal agencies aren't usually the best at cross-coordinating their related interactions with patients enrolled in the government health programs they individually administer. Exacerbating the malaise is the reality that patients often transition through multiple government-run health programs in their lifetime.

Worse yet, millions of patients concurrently enroll in two or more government-administered health programs.

While the best-known and extensively studied concurrent enrollments are of the vulnerable populations dually enrolled in the Medicare and Medicaid programs, the most complex concurrent enrollment scenarios occur with the veteran population.

Veterans, who have access to retiree military health benefits and veteran's health benefits, can sometimes find themselves concurrently enrolled in 4 or more government-administered health programs. Those health programs have significant amounts of benefit overlap and minimal cross-coordination or effective collaboration between program administrators.

As with the case of the Medicare program and VHA, veterans concurrently enrolled in both programs have significant overlap in covered benefits. Both programs serve as primary payers for those overlapping benefits. The benefit overlap and primary payer status create loopholes that American health care cartel members are adept at exploiting and converting into overpayments and overtreatments.

Those overpayments and overtreatments represent tens of billions of dollars in annual health care fraud, waste, and abuse. Health care fraud, waste, and abuse that members of the American health care cartel have become quite adept at laundering into "innovative" revenue growth and margin expansion.

I fundamentally believe there is no investment too significant to repay our nation's heroes for the sacrifice they and their families have made. However, the resulting impact of the overtreatments and overpayments that occur are negative externalities for veterans, their families, and taxpayers. With bigger budgets for federal agencies and higher revenues for American health care cartel members, many stakeholders involved in these transactions are satisfied with the status quo and current trends.

While leading the VA innovation center (VIC), I explored several pathways to closing existing loopholes. I facilitated several discussions with members of the leadership team at the CMS innovation center (CMMI). I met with Patrick Conway. Adam Boehler. Brad Smith. And career staff led by Arrah and Amy.

Unfortunately for American health care consumers and taxpayers, VA and CMSs' attempts to test approaches to closing some of those loopholes met with overwhelming resistance from agents of the American health care cartel.

I wasn't too surprised at the outcomes of VA's attempts to collaborate with CMS to test approaches that could reduce health care fraud, waste, and abuse.

The American health care cartel is mighty. The game is usually over once industrial complexes get in the mix.

For example, Congress eliminated the Chief Management Officer (CMO) role created at the Pentagon to pursue reforms. They did so after only a couple of years of its operation. A couple of years that resulted in Lisa Hershman, the Senate confirmed CMO, delivering Government Accountability Office (GAO) validated savings (mostly cost avoidance) over 37 billion dollars. However, according to the GAO report, the savings were not always well documented or consistent with the department's definitions of reform. Although the actual cost savings weren't 37 billion dollars, they weren't zero either.

While there were internal issues about the approach and tactics, the CMO's office achieved savings by eliminating billions in fraudulent, wasteful, and abusive spending, not by reducing the services, tools, or assets our warfighters needed to succeed.

As the Princeton economist Uwe Reinhardt said, "every dollar of health care spending is someone else's health care income, even when it's fraud, waste or abuse." The sentiment behind Uwe's statement applies to fraud, waste, and abuse in any context.

Anyone who attempts to take income away will face resistance and opposition. The savings the Pentagon created for taxpayers represented lost income for the military-industrial complex. A formidable opponent second only to the American health care industrial complex in its ability to pull levers that ensure its continued growth and success.

The military-industrial complex doesn't like to lose income. No one does. They eventually realized the CMO was generating savings for taxpayers. They put plans in motion to eliminate the additional authorities granted to the CMO. Although the CMO had different powers, the essential authority required to reform the Pentagon is the authority over appropriations.

If Congress appropriates a certain amount and purpose for spending, the staff or program office receiving those funds are required to obligate those funds as appropriated. A CMO empowered to root out fraud, waste, and abuse is thus "set up" to go against the will of Congress by challenging existing budget allocations and spending plans.

Unfortunately for taxpayers, the military-industrial complex was very effective in its quest to undermine a CMO's office designed to fail. Congress eliminated the CMO role and office in December 2020 with a 1-year sunset date. The military-industrial complex was exceptionally brazen with this initiative. They successfully compelled their allies in Congress to put a special provision into the bill that eliminated the Pentagon's CMO office.

The special provision prohibited anyone who had ever served as the Pentagon's CMO from managing any of the existing CMO's responsibilities during the sunset period. The inclusion of that language effectively prevented Lisa from being re-appointed by the Biden Administration. In case they were interested in doing that. The CMO's responsibilities were fragmented and distributed across different parts of the Pentagon.

Several federal health programs primarily function as purchasers. Some federal health programs like Medicare also act as payers. The Medicare program works directly with providers and producers to pay claims for services those providers and producers render to Medicare patients in its payer role.

Unfortunately, the majority of those transactions are fee-for-service transactions. The direct costs of the government administering health benefits in this manner are technically lower. However, there are several rules in place that prevent the government from aggressively addressing loopholes exploited when the fee-for-service approach pays providers and producers. The pervasiveness of those loopholes results in tens of billions of dollars in annual health care fraud, waste, and abuse.

Private payers have incentives to fight every claim and delay every payout to providers and producers.

Provider and producers are the stakeholders that render services to patients covered by the health benefit plans administered by the private payers.

The Affordable Care Act (ACA) and subsequent rules creating a floor for medical expenses as a percentage of premium revenues created a new challenge for private payers. A challenge they primarily chose to meet with increased industry consolidation.

With the enactment of new rules regarding medical expense minimums, a private payer seeking to maximize profit and shareholder returns could either grow by choosing to diversify its business or acquire other private payers. In a bid to increase revenues while contending with profit margin ceilings on revenues from premiums collected, most private payers focused on vertical and horizontal integration. In lay terms: they increased consolidation activities.

Physicians are the primary cohort authorized and licensed to deliver health care to patients in the American health care ecosystem. They are enabled to be the preeminent revenue-generating members of the provider community. Their position atop the revenue-generating hierarchy of the provider community has made establishing alliances with physicians or the acquisition of physicians essential to the growth strategy of stakeholders in the provider community.

Provider organizations like hospital-centric health systems can only survive if they are aligned with or control the dominant physicians in their coverage area. Without alignment with or control over physician behavior, most provider organizations cannot generate sufficient volumes to remain financially viable.

The current incentive model and other structural challenges to physicians remaining independent led to increasing consolidation and a rise in employed physicians over the last couple of decades. Physicians' loss of independence in medicine and health care delivery comes with its share of negative externalities to physicians and care teams.

Those negative externalities mainly manifest as increased physician and care team burnout, shorter patient visit times, and ever-increasing prices.

Producers manufacture and deliver goods and services. Those goods and services are considered interventions. Those interventions help providers care for patients or stay compliant with regulations. Those regulations govern the manufacturing and production processes of the goods and services used in the American health care ecosystem.

Producers organize and operate primarily based on how the regulatory bodies that authorize and license their activities permit them to organize and operate. As such, producers are the stakeholder group most incentivized to lobby regulators. Their lobbying helps make their pathways to profit maximization as easy as possible.

While producers have historically had to ally with provider organizations and physicians to get their products and services adopted by patients, producers have significantly increased direct patient engagement without the primary providers' consent. To combat this trend, providers often lobby regulators to restrict the types of products and services patients can consume without their permission.

Certain pharmaceuticals, medical devices and supplies, and technology interventions are sometimes only accessible to patients with the consent of their physician or provider representative. While restricting patient access to some specific interventions is prudent, there are many scenarios where the benign nature of the intervention shouldn't require provider engagement before consumption.

However, because producers have significant incentives to exploit patients to boost revenues, regulators thought it prudent to route most patients' access to reimbursable products and services through their primary care provider.

Though prudent, the forced inclusion of providers in most of the interactions patients have with producers has contributed to the increasing complexity and cost of the functioning of the American health care ecosystem.

When one considers how complex, expensive, and inequitable the American health care ecosystem is, the roles and incentives of the different key stakeholders are a powerful driving force behind the functioning of the current American health care ecosystem.

There are several reasons why the current key stakeholders have the roles they have. The COVID-19 pandemic made it clear that while several stakeholders are vital to the functioning of the current health care ecosystem, not all current "key" stakeholders are essential.

Exacerbating this crisis is the reality that not all essential stakeholders are empowered to be key stakeholders. Many critical stakeholders don't have a say or sufficient leverage to ensure adequate resolution of concerns they raise. As concerns of essential workers remain unaddressed, the American health care ecosystem continues to achieve mediocre outcomes while undermining American prosperity.

To actualize the simple, affordable, and equitable American health care ecosystem we need, <u>essential stakeholders must be the key stakeholders with the loudest voices and most leverage</u> during health reform negotiations.

That's the truth.

The whole truth.

Nothing but the truth.

Key Drivers of High Costs and Health Spending

"Every penny of fraud, waste, and abuse is someone's income. Expect them to put up a fight if you attempt to take it away."

The costs of delivering health services are determined by market dynamics in different states and counties across the nation and influenced by government regulations. Further, the incentives inherent to fee-for-service payment models and legacy technology infrastructure enable the complexity, high prices, and increasing spending that is pervasive across the American health care industry.

The market dynamics of different states and counties across America and the overall health and well-being of the residents of the respective states lead to significant variation in costs and prices of health care goods and services sold in each state. The resulting variance in costs and prices leads to different consumption patterns by the residents of each state. According to Kaiser Family Foundation (KFF) analysis, in 2014, U.S. health spending per capita was 8,045 dollars, with two states exceeding eleven thousand dollars per capita. The District of Columbia, which isn't a state, is an outlier with 11,944 dollars per capita health spending. According to the same KFF analysis, in 2014, Alaska was the state with the highest per capita spending. Alaska's per capita spending was 11,064 dollars in 2014. According to the same KFF analysis, the state with the lowest per capita health spending in 2014 was Utah, which came at 5,982 dollars that year.

According to a recent analysis completed and published by the Health Care Cost Institute (HCCI) across counties and metro areas in the U.S., they saw up to 25-fold variation in median prices of the same services. For example, the median price for C-sections in some parts of California was nearly 4.5

times the prices paid in parts of Tennessee. Standard blood tests in parts of Texas were priced at almost 25 times the prices paid for the same blood test in parts of Ohio. Finally, office visits, one of the most common services offered, were priced in different parts of Alaska at 3-times the prices paid for the same service in parts of Florida.

Variances in cost and price lead many patients to seek certain types of care outside their home state and even outside the nation. With pricing and variance for some high-cost procedures being exorbitantly high, patients realize they can still come out ahead on how much they spend if they travel to a higher-value state to receive specific health care services. That is usually more prudent versus staying local and paying exorbitant prices. According to The American Journal of Medicine, in 2017, more than 1.4 million Americans sought health care in various countries worldwide. The most common reason more Americans have become medical tourists is that they desire less expensive health care.

While there are many reasons for high health care costs and spending, one of the most prevalent reasons for increased costs in a specific state is how consolidated and powerful American health care cartel members are in any particular state.

A variety of factors drive spending, including rates of insurance coverage and accessibility of providers. With insurance coverage and accessibility, patients seek care when they need it. Providers encourage patients to consume as much reimbursable medically necessary care as they can, most of the time. Some bad actors remove "medically necessary" from their lexicon.

In addition to market consolidation and patient needs driving high costs and spending, one additional key driver is how well social drivers of health like nutrition, educational attainment, exercise, etcetera are tended to by state and county governments. The main driver exacerbating all the aforementioned key drivers is the prevalence of unaddressed mental illness or behavioral health issues in the population of any state.

In addition to market consolidation, the patient's needs, unaddressed social drivers of health and mental illness drive costs and spending higher. Also, the complexity of the American health care ecosystem introduces significant opacity to the process, worsening the situation. Complexities in the American health care ecosystem persist because the American health care cartel continues to resist attempts to introduce transparency and accountability.

Transparency remains challenging to introduce because American health care ecosystem transactions remain beholden to legacy fee-for-service architecture. Bolstering those transactions are byzantine diagnosis codes, billing codes and rules, and a laundry list of other regulatory requirements for operating and transacting in the American health care ecosystem. That complexity adds another layer of costs. Those costs evolve into overhead costs for American health care ecosystem stakeholders.

While the promise of consolidation has been better integration, more efficiency, and higher quality, consolidation has only delivered a more consolidated health care ecosystem with mostly higher prices. Those higher prices are increasingly shifting to patients and health care consumers.

Markets with the worst dynamics either have a combination of a high concentration of providers and a low concentration of payers or a high concentration of payers and a low concentration of providers. In either scenario, the stakeholder with the higher concentration has more negotiating leverage and dictates the terms of engagement. The worst scenario that leads to the highest prices is a high concentration of providers and a low payer concentration. In such a scenario, the provider charges exorbitant fees, which lead to higher premiums. In markets with high payer concentration and low provider concentration, even though the payer has more leverage, the payer cannot dictate unsustainably low prices to the providers. Payers need to have a network of providers to market and sell to purchasers. Providers can opt-out of working with payers altogether and establish direct contracting relationships with patients and purchasers alike.

While price controls have been discussed and entertained, the American health care cartel has ensured such discussions didn't get much traction. In another show of force and greed, the American health care cartel put rules in place to limit the ability of the largest federal government payer to negotiate for certain goods and services that are paid for by the federal government.

This malaise is evident in the federal government's inability to negotiate for prescription drugs reimbursed by Medicare Part D. According to Kaiser Family Foundation, Medicare Part D is a voluntary outpatient prescription drug benefit for people with Medicare, provided through private plans approved by the federal government. The Congressional Budget Office (CBO) estimates that spending on Part D benefits will total 96 billion dollars in 2021. While the federal government spends tens of billions of dollars a year on prescription drugs, the American health care cartel ensures that its members included those transactions get to dictate whatever prices they want to the federal government buyer.

Those prices have steadily increased over time.

Costs, prices, and spending are on the rise as market dynamics worsen. The American health care cartels' desire to sustain revenues and profit by acquiring sufficient leverage to demand higher fees is fueling this malaise. Payers have consolidated in recent years and are also aggressively pursuing a vertical integration strategy by acquiring their provider partners. UnitedHealth Group has been the most prolific of the group and the largest payvider organization in America. Probably the world.

The merger of CVS Health and Aetna demonstrates alternative approaches pursued to establish a powerful, far-reaching payvider organization.

Adding to this consolidation trend has been the significant uptick in hospital mergers and the surge in hospital-owned physician practices. As hospitals consolidated over the years and dramatically increased the number of physician practices they controlled, the pseudo-monopolies and actual monopolies that were created caused a dramatic increase in prices. Those excessive price increases occur in states and regional markets where the hospital-owned physician practices were the most dominant.

With the costs and risks of owning an independent practice rising every year, the government exacerbates the challenges independent physician practices contend with by increasing their regulatory burden and preferentially providing financial aid to hospital-centric provider organizations. For example, during the COVID-19 pandemic, hospitals received most of the federal funding directed at the provider community. While patients needed intensive care and many were cared for in hospitals, many patients received care in the community. That care prevented many from needing to go to the hospital. Worse yet, many hospital-centric provider organizations used their COVID-19 relief funds from the government to acquire other physician groups and Ambulatory Surgical Centers (ASCs). It would appear that the deck is increasingly stacked against physician independence. It is. That is the American health care cartels' focus at the moment.

While many were being cared for in the community, hundreds of thousands were deteriorating and dying at home.

The people that deteriorated and died in their homes didn't receive any care from hospitals that received most of the funding designated for care delivery during the pandemic.

The structure of the American health care ecosystem, related fee-for-service transaction fund flows, and the ability of the American health care cartel to manipulate American health care markets to their benefit creates a lot of excess cost and waste. The primary drivers of that waste are failures of care delivery, care coordination, and pricing failures. Worsening these primary drivers of waste are overtreatment, administrative complexity, fraud, and abuse.

Addressing these festering drivers of waste can only occur if we reform campaign finance corruption, partisan gerrymandering, and voter suppression laws.

The American health care ecosystem, as currently designed, is incentivized to enable failures of care delivery.

Failures of care delivery primarily occur when care delivery systems fail to deliver the best care to patients or follow leading evidence-based practices when caring for patients. This type of failure often causes worse patient outcomes and higher costs for the American health care ecosystem. The American health care cartel profits from the higher prices and recurring revenues from patients whose poor clinical outcomes from a failed encounter deteriorate into chronic pain or illness.

Failures of care coordination are similar to failures of care delivery but tend to be more overt and in line with the stated policy of care delivery organizations. Failures of care coordination usually occur when providers who are incentivized not to collaborate with other providers caring for the same patient refuse to do so or choose to collaborate in a delayed manner.

By refusing to share information or effectively supporting a patient's journey to engage external providers, some providers explicitly undermine a patient's ability to achieve optimal health outcomes. This harsh reality exists and remains pervasive because those providers have low or negative incentives to improve care coordination for patients seeking care from external providers.

Some care delivery organizations like hospital-centric health systems have stringent and explicit rules about sharing patient information with external provider groups. Those care delivery organizations are adept at making it challenging for patients or external provider groups to transmit or receive patient data. That information is necessary for the external provider group to understand the patient's history or provide higher-value care. This practice is known as information blocking, and it wastes everyone's time, resources, and empathy.

The most common tactic includes requiring patients to pay fees to receive a copy of their health records, a financial barrier for many lower-income patients. Transmitting paper records, either by fax or handing a printed copy to patients, delaying the length of time before the information is shared, and sharing the information in hard-to-use formats are some of the other tactics used.

The lack of transparency enabled by fee-for-service transactions and related legacy technology facilitating fund flows is the underlying reason for pricing failures in the American health care ecosystem. These pricing failures and the resulting information asymmetry allow the American health care cartel to maximize opportunities to capture economic rents.

The American health care cartel can maximize economic rents as those pricing failures persist. They aggressively oppose attempts to implement regulatory changes designed to address pricing failures. The regulations that promote price transparency, reference pricing, price controls, and related approaches designed to resolve pricing failures meet overwhelming resistance.

Overwhelming resistance typically manifests as lobbying efforts to kill, weaken, or pivot regulatory actions to reduce or eliminate pricing failures.

Overtreatment is pervasive across the American health care ecosystem. It persists because many key stakeholders have incentives to seek or deliver more care. Once patients lose their motivation to primarily consume higher-value care, they expand their appetite for care. They proactively seek to consume as much care as they are legally allowed.

Some patients suffer from unaddressed behavioral health issues. For those patients, legal limits usually don't apply. Those patients often pursue fraudulent means to acquiring access to care options and interventions they may have gotten addicted to during their encounters with the American health care ecosystem. The American health care cartel enables such addiction.

Ubiquitous fee-for-service payment models incentivize both providers and producers to deliver higher volumes of their goods and services. Those higher volumes are known to exceed amounts that are medically indicated or beneficial to a patient's well-being. This practice persists because the delivery of higher volumes of goods and services allows provider and producer members of the American health care cartel to maximize the economic rents they extract from the American health care ecosystem.

Fee-for-service payment models and the legacy technology systems or intermediaries that enable them often bake administrative complexity into the American health care ecosystem.

The administrative complexity enabled by fee-for-service payment models is exacerbated by the regulations, contracting peculiarities, and market dynamics governing the execution of those fee-for-service transactions.

Increasing administrative complexity usually translates to American health care ecosystem stakeholders requiring the services of esoteric knowledge experts.

Those esoteric knowledge experts are usually costly to employ or retain since their knowledge is highly specialized. Most opt to rent them instead. Their knowledge has limited intrinsic value. It is deemed valuable primarily because of the idiosyncrasies of changing reimbursement regulations, fee-for-service transactions, and related fund flows.

The armies of lawyers, consultants, financial professionals, health economists, and former regulators that earn a living as esoteric knowledge experts in the American health care industry have incentives to lobby for increased administrative complexity. That additional administrative complexity allows them to increase their rates and maximize opportunities to extract economic rents from the American health care ecosystem.

The idiosyncrasies of fee-for-service transactions and key stakeholder incentives create ample opportunity for fraud and abuse. There are thousands of regulations, rules, and tools designed to limit or eliminate fraud and abuse. Unfortunately, the American health care cartel enables the design of loopholes into the implemented regulations, rules, and tools, allowing existing or new examples of fraud and abuse to grow.

While there are far-ranging estimates of the impact of fraud and abuse across the American health care industry, the federal government typically collects billions of dollars in fines while prosecuting thousands of offenders every year. However, the federal government still loses hundreds of billions of taxpayer funds. The American health care cartel always wins. Always.

The American health care cartel has incentives to enable and scale drivers of excess cost and waste across the American health care ecosystem. They can only continue to do so because of campaign finance corruption, partisan gerrymandering, and voter suppression laws.

Several health care consumers and taxpayers are aware of many of the tactics mentioned above. They have often rallied to try and overcome the cartel's opposition to change. Their efforts have had minimal impact because of campaign finance corruption, partisan gerrymandering, and voter suppression laws.

Resolving the drivers of excess cost and waste is the most significant opportunity to increase the value of the American health care ecosystem.

We can only resolve the drivers of excess cost and waste if we reform campaign finance corruption, partisan gerrymandering, and voter suppression laws.

That's the truth.

The whole truth.

Nothing but the truth.

Health Reform

"We have never seen health as a right. It has been conceived as a privilege, available only to those who can afford it. This is the real reason the American health care system is in such a scandalous state."
— Rep. Shirley Chisholm

While eliminating excess cost can improve the system, only the right incentives, regulations, and tools will enable key stakeholders to pursue this path. The method of payment determines which stakeholder group gets the savings from waste reduction. As such, key stakeholders who can't get savings from waste reduction efforts will resist implementing such measures.

In addition to the fee-for-service approach to executing payment transactions and fund flows, "alternative" payment models have been designed and tested. Although "alternative" payment models technically exist based on the nature of the contractual agreement between transacting stakeholders, most of those "alternative" payment models are built on technically complex fee-for-service transaction architecture and related legacy technology. The ensuing marriage between fee-for-service payment models and "alternative" payment models automatically converts "alternative" payment models to supplemental payment models. Supplemental because it is a derivative of the existing fee-for-service model. It doesn't give stakeholders an actual alternative to utilizing fee-for-service transaction architecture and legacy technology systems or intermediaries.

Exacerbating the technical challenges associated with executing the "alternative" payment models is the reality that those "alternative" payment models are still subject to many of the complexities, constraints, and challenges of fee-for-service transactions.

Esoteric knowledge experts are one of the primary beneficiaries of "alternative" payment models because its evolution introduces additional complexity to the existing complexity of fee-for-service transactions.

Fee-for-service transaction architecture undergirds cost-plus payment models, episode-based payment models, and population-based payment models often viewed as "alternatives." The most prevalent payment models put the savings with payers who aren't well-positioned to develop and implement meaningful waste-reducing, quality improvement initiatives at the provider organizations they contract or partner with.

In a cost-plus payment model, payers contract with providers for their services based on what it actually costs the provider to deliver the service unit plus a mutually agreed-upon profit margin. While this model is relatively straightforward to implement and may even be designed without reliance on fee-for-service transaction architecture, only payers stand to gain if any savings are generated using this approach. As such, providers are reticent to adopt cost-plus payment models because they have no financial incentive to do so.

Episode-based payment models bundle a set of services at a pre-negotiated price for the bundled services. Some episode-based payments also have bonuses or penalties attached. Those bonuses or penalties are realized based on the outcomes of specific episodes of care. Both payers and providers stand to benefit from different types of savings achieved while utilizing episode-based payments. There have been more successful attempts over the years and several rounds of health reform activities to implement various episode-based payment models. Episode-based payment models have been adopted at a reasonable scale. However, the American health care cartel ensures that the current approach to adopting episode-based payment models results in additional complexity, cost, and inequities across the American health care ecosystem.

Population-based payments are the only type of payments that reward providers with savings generated from reducing all the different types of waste in the American health care ecosystem. With population-based payment models, providers have incentives to reduce operational inefficiencies, unnecessary care delivery, and unnecessary encounters with patients. Though incentivized, several factors limit the effective and sustainable delivery of services under population-based payment models. There have been ongoing attempts to reform the American health care ecosystem to embrace population-based payment models. The American health care cartel primarily leads those ongoing attempts. This unfortunate reality results in increasing complexity, cost, and inequities associated with implementing and scaling population-based payment models. Although ongoing reform efforts are significant, they have often generated minimal savings because those measures are often designed to pursue different objectives and spread across multiple uncoordinated entities. This flawed tactical approach to reform ensures increased costs and complexity are a mainstay.

With a stated mandate to reduce waste, reform efforts pursue the Triple Aim by moving from volume-based, fee-for-service clinical delivery and payment to value-based models. Volume-based models utilize fee-for-service payment models that incentivize higher volumes of care that focus on maximizing revenue from specific encounters. Value-based models use outcomes-based payments that incentivize better care delivery focused on improving patients' long-term health and well-being. Volume-based care delivery is notorious for incentivizing providers to only focus on individual interactions and encounters with patients while utilizing retrospective information to facilitate the conversation.

On the other hand, value-based care delivery incentivizes providers to embrace a team-based care continuum that promotes collaboration and coordination across all the providers involved in the care of a single patient. Value-based care delivery has incentives to develop processes and adopt tools that enable predictive use of information.

The Triple Aim is a framework developed by the Institute for Healthcare Improvement (IHI) to assist health care systems in optimizing performance, reducing costs, and improving patient care through various interventions and metrics. Since Triple Aim goals were first defined and publicized in 2007, the construct has caught on with the emergence of quadruple aims and even quintuple aims. While additional aims have emerged over the years, sustainably or systematically achieving any of those aims remains elusive across the American health care ecosystem.

While several different combinations and words describe the Triple Aim, widely accepted constructs have defined the Triple Aim as improving health, reducing cost, and improving quality. While lowering costs should be relatively straightforward to define and calculate, the fee-for-service architecture that undergirds most implemented value-based payment models makes it challenging for stakeholders to determine, calculate, or reduce costs.

Efforts to improve health or quality come with some unique challenges. Improving health can be challenging because optimal health means different things to different people and organizations. The design of the American health care ecosystem primarily seeks to care for the sick. The ecosystem doesn't have incentives to promote public health. Its design doesn't enable it to engage people about adopting healthy behaviors. Improving quality can be even more challenging because there is no consensus across the American health care ecosystem about what quality is, which quality measures should be considered preeminent, and how quality measures should be captured and reported.

Defining, prioritizing, and evaluating quality has become such a complicated endeavor that many stakeholders have started shifting their vocabulary and focus towards improving patient experience as their preferred third aim. Others have chosen to tack on experience as a fourth aim. Those that choose to pursue a fifth aim tend to include access to care as the fifth aim.

Movement from fee-for-service to value-based payment and clinical delivery has been slow and limited by significant barriers to health service providers sustaining revenues and increasing accountability for patient outcomes.

It would appear logical to hold providers accountable for the health outcomes their patients achieve. However, providers are reticent to take on that responsibility because they are acutely aware of the limited impact access to medical service delivery has on improving health outcomes.

Social drivers of health have a more significant impact on health outcomes.

Incumbents are ill-equipped to address social drivers of health. And many don't want to.

Let's imagine a world where the American health care cartel stops resisting reform efforts. <u>Unlikely, but let's step into fantasyland for a minute</u>.

Successful pursuit of the Triple Aim will require the creation and testing of innovative care delivery models. Paradigm-shifting models that focus more on improving the health and well-being of communities of people. Efforts that focus on building the reimagined infrastructure needed to manage care across modalities and sites of care successfully. Care is coordinated over time and across several independent organizations.

Improving the health and well-being of communities starts with stratifying or segmenting populations in those communities based on health and well-being status and needs.

Once stratified, at-risk or rising risk populations should be targeted with interventions designed to improve their health while reducing costs. Pursuing the Triple Aim requires providers to adopt structures and processes that enable Population Health Management (PHM) while transitioning from fee-for-service payment models.

PHM is a core competency for providers in a non-fee-for-service environment. Its adoption by providers is essential to a meaningful shift to a value-based health care ecosystem. While crucial, reimbursement for PHM activities isn't currently richly rewarded. As such, providers often balance how to optimize performance and maximize economic rents in the current environment. They do this while figuring out the optimal moment to commit to the value-based payment movement.

The prevailing narrative remains that a departure from fee-for-service is inevitable. It isn't. Yes. Fee-for-service reimbursement rates are often growing at rates lower than inflation. The American health care cartel doesn't care. Its provider members are doubling down on fee-for-service payment models. They are simply pursuing tactics to improve the productivity of their employed care teams. Those tactics usually manifest as shortened visit times, smaller care teams, and increasingly frustrated patients and care teams.

With any transition or modernization effort, coordination, change management, and new tools enable success. PHM is no different in that regard. Population health strategies focused on care coordination and care team cohesion are vital. Pursuit of such techniques will likely motivate providers to adopt new tools designed to analyze the panel of patients in their care. Ideally, once target panels of patients are selected, those new tools identify care gaps, stratify risks, engage patients, manage care, and measure outcomes.

With the adoption of new tools, providers also have to invest in effective change management to ensure that the transition from fee-for-service to value-based payment models is as frictionless as possible.

The design of any value-based payment model is essential to its ability to incentivize the pursuit of the Triple Aim.

With effectively designed value-based payment models, providers have incentives to use new tools to augment the role of their care teams, effectively engage their patient populations, achieve better health outcomes, and decrease overall costs.

<u>Fantasy time over</u>.

The American health care cartel won't allow anything I described to happen at scale.

They're adept at running charades and elevating manicured talking points.

Fundamental change isn't happening. The cartel won't allow it. Like parasites embracing its host, they go along till they figure out how to kill or maim the "innovative" new fad proclaimed as the panacea that will "fix" American health care.

AMERICAN HEALTH CARE ISN'T BROKEN!

You can't fix things that aren't broken.

Only broken things can be fixed.

While there is some desire for a shift to value-based payment models, concerns persist, limiting adoption. Concerns about methods used for measuring health outcomes are some of the typical concerns raised. Stakeholder concerns about their ability to unilaterally control costs and make more money by adopting value-based payment models remain central to the resistance. In reality, most of the concerns that persist arise primarily because American health care ecosystem stakeholders know the rules of the game and recognize the outsized influence American health care cartel members have on how the health care industry functions.

The American health care cartel has little incentive to support the transition from fee-for-service payments to value-based payment models.

This reality comes as no surprise since institutions and organizations function as designed and incentivized. This reality results in the limited adoption of effective value-based payment models disconnected from fee-for-service transaction architecture.

Members of the American health care cartel often lend lip service and present the façade that they are proactively pursuing effective value-based payment models. Some survey results even reflect significant support for a switch to value-based models.

Unfortunately for the health care consumer, the American health care cartel has been mainly smoke and mirrors with no tangible actions to back it up.

In the decade since the enactment of the Affordable Care Act (ACA) that codified several of the tenets of the desired shift to value-based payment models, most American health care ecosystem transactions are still facilitated using fee-for-service contracts and transaction architecture.

Many providers and payers proclaimed they were "all in." They received additional funding to make required investments in tools and resources to aid in their transitions. Most providers and payers failed to achieve any meaningful adoption of value-based payment models.

Value-based models disconnected from fee-for-service transaction architecture are scarce. Unicorns.

In addition to overwhelming resistance from members of the American health care cartel, several complicating factors contribute to the limited effectiveness of efforts to transform the American health care ecosystem.

First, several technical, policy, political, and market barriers obstruct critical pathways to system-wide adoption of effective value-based models.

Second, key stakeholders often employ the tactic of avoiding being accountable for complex populations. In contrast, many stakeholders shift the costs to others instead of pursuing strategies capable of eliminating certain expenses.

Third, dominant groups, primarily members of the American health care cartel, create market dynamics that limit the value realized from payment and care delivery reform efforts.

Fourth, persistent structural and cultural barriers to system-wide adherence to leading clinical practices even in cases where incentives are aligned to enable adoption.

Given the pervasiveness of the aforementioned complicating factors, a comprehensive understanding of underlying key issues causing these complicating factors will highlight opportunities for consumers of American health care to resolve them and effectively pursue systemic, lasting change.

Barriers Obstructing Critical Pathways

"There are no constraints on the human mind, no walls around the human spirit, and no barriers to our progress, except those we ourselves erect." – President Ronald Reagan

Regulatory and or technical barriers diminish or eliminate profit or revenue-enhancing business cases that enable key stakeholder adoption of effective solutions. The American health care cartel facilitated the design and implementation of the Affordable Care Act (ACA). They didn't engage with any intention of achieving many of the stated objectives of the ACA. While affordable care was the stated objective, the jury is in. American health care is no more affordable for American society today than before the ACA became law.

In many instances, it's a lot less affordable for many individuals, businesses, states, and the federal government. While there are many reasons the ACA failed to achieve its stated objective of affordability, it did manage to achieve its unstated aim of being a jobs program and channel to funnel more taxpayer funds to the American health care cartel. Taxpayer funds that primarily manifested as unsustainable subsidies designed to shift the cost of running the American health care ecosystem to taxpayers without any requirements to meaningfully reduce the costs and spending of the American health care ecosystem.

Like most poorly designed efforts, stated objectives and desired outcomes are meaningless. The dirt, as they say, is in the details. The truth is revealed in the outcomes achieved and solutions excluded from consideration during conversations about reform. The ACA was no different because the American health care cartel ensured that its heart's desire was what manifested with the enactment of the ACA. The American health care cartel's heart desire isn't aligned with the stated objective of the ACA. A stated goal to usher in an era of affordable health care for all.

Barely a couple of years after enacting the ACA, American health care cartel members started abandoning ACA programs they had previously committed to. They also quickly shifted to a harshly critical tone. The American health care cartel became emboldened and increased their criticism of the ACA, especially after the Democrats lost their majority in the House of Representatives (The House) to the Republicans during the mid-term elections during the first term of the Obama Administration. The Obama Administration spent almost all of its goodwill and political capital contorting itself in futile efforts to acquiesce to demands that Republican and independent Senators had of the ACA. Unfortunately for Democrats, they still had to enact the ACA with no Republican votes after agreeing to several convoluted compromises.

Optimistically, given the benefit of knowing what they know now, I assume Democrats will pursue a different approach next time they can unilaterally enact sweeping changes to the American health care ecosystem.

Hopefully, their chosen approach results in a paradigm-shift, assuming the American health care cartel allows that to happen. Unlikely.

One of the most challenging barriers to advancing the transition to value-based payments is the ongoing, system-wide investment in tools, resources, intermediaries, and technologies designed to facilitate complicated fee-for-service transactions.

Those assets have become the lifeblood and defense mechanism for most providers and payers in the American health care industry.

For providers, the tools and technologies they have adopted to facilitate their fee-for-service transactions are also where they retain patient and clinical practice information. They use the patient and clinical practice information to their advantage in negotiations or information blocking schemes.

While the concept of Electronic Health Records (EHRs) technically makes sense, the pathway the American health care cartel insisted EHR evolution should follow ensured that incumbent EHR suppliers maintained control of the EHR market.

EHR supplier members of the American health care cartel are notorious for malfeasance that delays effective Revenue Cycle Management (RCM) of fee-for-service transactions for any providers that attempt to move away from fee-for-service transaction architecture.

Further, with the enactment of the ACA, the American health care cartel ensured that providers were required to adopt certified EHRs. Adhering to the requirements of certification primarily written by incumbent EHR suppliers usually meant that new entrants in the EHR arena essentially had to build complex and expensive solutions. Most of those solutions are merely putting a fancy veneer on an architecture designed to facilitate fee-for-service transactions.

For payers, the tools and technologies they have adopted to facilitate fee-for-service transactions serve as a data moat that allows them to resist attempts at reform or intrusion on their territory by any new, disruptive entrant. The information asymmetry enabled by their data moat grants most payers the competitive edge in contracting negotiations with other American health care cartel members.

Both payer and EHR supplier members of the American health care cartel uniquely benefit from their existing investments in legacy tools and technologies. Those assets are designed to facilitate fee-for-service transactions. They are usually in cahoots in quelling attempts to move away from fee-for-service transaction architecture.

In addition to barriers specific to adopting value-based payment models disconnected from fee-for-service transaction architecture, adopting most information technology solutions is often fraught with significant challenges. Those significant challenges take various forms. Interoperability challenges often prove insurmountable to adoption. Any new information technology solution is typically required to exchange information with the legacy tools and technologies it seeks to replace or additional tools and technologies the provider intends to maintain.

Interoperability with other vendor systems usually presents the most significant challenges since many information technology vendors aren't in the habit of building solutions that make it convenient for providers to work with multiple vendors. Most information technology vendors that service providers prefer to sell a suite of solutions designed to fulfill as many RCM requirements that a provider might have. This go-to-market approach employed by EHR suppliers intends to preclude any disruptive new entrant from gaining a toehold with a provider.

Even when new entrants manage to gain a toehold with a provider, those providers are conditioned to quickly usher the potentially disruptive new entrant to integrate their solution with the provider's EHR platform. Those integration marathons are often laden with additional costs, delays, and sabotage designed to frustrate potentially disruptive new entrants seeking to deploy their solution at the provider organization. While many disruptive new entrants run out of money or go out of business wading through the muck of EHR integration marathons, others have their technology or "secret sauce" stolen by EHR suppliers and adapted into the incumbents' EHR application. Once the incumbents' EHR application updates their platform with features offered by the new entrant, the EHR supplier excludes the new entrant from working with the provider. They often inform the provider that they were "unable to integrate" the potentially disruptive new entrants solution into their EHR platform. They offer the consolation prize of a couple of updated features they have introduced into the EHR platform. Those updated features are usually cost an arm and a leg.

Beyond interoperability challenges, human and cost-related challenges also hinder the adoption of new information technology solutions. The employees at a provider organization have typically gotten used to working with legacy technology solutions and usually don't have the requisite skills to use new information technology systems. In such scenarios, in addition to the cost and time required to train employees on how to use the updated information technology solutions, providers often have to contend with employees that are incapable or unwilling to adapt to new, technology-enabled approaches to performing their duties.

In addition to the presence of skills gaps, other human challenges exist. Some of those other human challenges are related to achieving consensus on required data standards, protocols, and formats. The challenges mentioned above usually slow or end provider organization efforts to adopt new information technology solutions.

Cost and sustainable approaches to generating cost savings are typically also barriers hindering the adoption of new information technology. In addition, some jobs usually performed by humans get eliminated when the adoption of new information technology enables digital transformation and automation. Accordingly, rationalizing development costs and identifying viable approaches to generating cost savings are usually crucial challenges providers must overcome when adopting new information technology.

Providers have to contend with several categories of cost when evaluating whether or not they should adopt new information technology. Direct costs include purchasing costs, annual maintenance costs, financing costs, and costs of supportive infrastructure required to operate the new information technology system. Supportive infrastructure costs are typically directed towards upgrades to hardware and physical spaces or expanding internet bandwidth. Indirect costs include but aren't limited to productivity loss, employee upskilling, and the level of effort required to evaluate and select a new information technology system.

Most employees are wary of the impact on workflows and job security of adopting new information technology solutions. As such, most provider organizations typically face employee resistance to the adoption of new information technology solutions. As provider organizations evaluate EHR and other technology solutions that may meet their needs, those efforts typically meet resistance from employees who don't want to change work habits. The opposition often makes it challenging to reach a consensus within the provider organization. An agreement that's usually required to achieve approval and eventually adoption of a new information technology system.

In addition to regulatory and technical barriers, provider appetite for and ability to manage risk has resulted in many value-based payment models retaining fee-for-service transaction architecture. The Centers for Medicare and Medicaid Services (CMS) set a goal of shifting more than 50-percent of Medicare fee-for-service payments to Alternative Payment Models (APMs) within the first 10-years of the enactment of the ACA. Unfortunately, almost all the APMs they decided to test ultimately retained fee-for-service transaction architecture. In reality, most of the APMs in circulation are actually supplemental payment models. They are primarily connected to fee-for-service architecture. By maintaining fee-for-service transaction architecture, the vast majority of the APMs CMS touts as essential to its transition from fee-for-service, essentially retained all the complexities of fee-for-service transactions while further complicating fund flows with idiosyncrasies of APMs. Costs associated with implementing some of those additional complexities usually eliminated most of the cost-savings expected from the adoption of APMs.

According to the value-based payment taxonomy created by CMS, the shift from fee-for-service to population-based payments occurs across four categories. The first category is traditional fee-for-service payments, and the fourth category is population-based payments. With the first category, payments are driven by the volume of services with no link to quality or efficiency. With the fourth category, payment isn't explicitly linked to the delivery of services, so the completion of any specific service doesn't trigger payment. Instead, payments in the fourth category are paid to clinicians and provider organizations over an extended period. An extended period that supposedly empowers clinicians and provider organizations with the time and financial incentives to pursue the best health outcomes for their patients.

The second category of the taxonomy is fee-for-service linked to quality. With the second category, some payment changes rely on the quality or efficiency of the care delivered to the patient. The payment changes are considered bonuses or penalties. With the third category, APMs built on fee-for-service architecture are the norm. Payments in this category are expected to be linked to effective management of populations or episodes of care. While payments in the third category remain triggered by the delivery of services, opportunities for two-sided risk or shared savings exist.

To achieve shared savings or enter into two-sided risk contracts with CMS, provider organizations formed Accountable Care Organizations (ACOs). According to CMS, an ACO is a coordinated organization of health care practitioners who agree to be accountable for the quality, cost, and overall care of Medicare beneficiaries enrolled in the traditional fee-for-service program. Medicare enrollees attributed to the ACO.

The term Accountable Care Organization was brought into the mainstream by Elliott Fisher in 2006 during a discussion of the Medicare Payment Advisory Commission (MedPAC). MedPAC is an independent, non-partisan legislative branch agency established to advise Congress on the administration of the Medicare program. MedPAC's mandate is broad enough to evaluate a wide range of issues affecting the Medicare program.

The creation of new entities labeled ACOs was part of the ACA. ACO advocates established trade associations like the National Association of Accountable Care Organizations (NAACOs) and technology-enablement companies like Aledade.

My initial encounter with the founder of Aledade, Farzad Mostashari, was in the summer of 2016. At the time, Aledade was barely two years old. He founded Aledade and successfully raised tens of millions of dollars of startup capital from Venture Capital firms. Farzad was also one of the many architects of the ACA alongside one of Aledade's lead investors, Bob Kocher, an investor at Venrock Capital.

I was still in my role at the Laura and John Arnold Foundation at the time. He was trying to sell me on a concept (something related to increasing borrowing costs for hospitals to reduce their incentive to pursue capital-intensive building expansion projects) he wanted me to share with John Arnold. I told him the concept was likely outside our grant-making scope, and I didn't think John would be interested in pursuing the idea personally.

When we spoke, I let him know I didn't think ACOs were designed or positioned meaningfully to bend the health care cost curve. He didn't like hearing that. At all. Whether attempting to lower costs across the American health care ecosystem or improving quality, ACOs can't defeat the American health care cartel.

I explained to him how even if physician-led ACOs reduced hospital utilization, those hospitals with reduced utilization still have market power sufficient to extract higher fees from commercially insured health benefit plans. Those hospitals will eventually hire, acquire or form Joint Ventures (JVs) with the physicians leading those ACOs. I also let him know that those independent physicians will ultimately succumb to the significant challenges associated with independent practice ownership and the allure of higher compensation associated with being a hospital-owned physician group.

I went on to share a concept I thought could become viable at scale. The idea I shared with Farzad was a combination of Professor Michael Porter's Centers-of-Excellence (CoE) strategy and medical tourism. He said he thought it was interesting, but he was focusing on building Aledade and didn't have the capacity or interest in pursuing anything else at the time. A few weeks after our conversation, the Dartmouth ACO announced that they were dropping out of Medicare's ACO program. Dartmouth's ACO cited mounting financial losses from their participation in the ACO program. Dartmouth's decision to drop out sent shockwaves across the ACO market because researchers at Dartmouth College developed the ACO model that was enacted by the ACA.

The most infuriating barrier obstructing critical pathways to improved health outcomes is that effective solutions designed to address the needs of the costliest chronically ill patients haven't been prioritized or enacted by recent health reform legislation. Even when enacted legislation can address the needs of the most expensive chronically ill patients, the American health care cartel undermines its implementation. There are many examples of provisions of the ACA that weren't implemented correctly or at all. Cases of final regulations not being enforced also highlight the reality that even after legislation and regulations are approved by the President of the United States or Cabinet members leading federal agencies, the American health care cartel can undermine the implementation of those efforts.

Chronically ill persons with functional limitations and mental illness are the costliest chronically ill patients served by the American health care ecosystem. Some state's resistance to Medicaid expansion limits access to care for functionally limited people and the mentally ill. Those same states are the first to complain about having insufficient resources to address the mental health care needs or Long Term Services and Supports (LTSS) requirements of their residents.

The design and function of the Medicaid program incentivize state governments to worsen health disparities for millions of Americans who rely on the program.

Those disparities are most harmful to mothers and infants.

That reality is reprehensible.

We must improve it.

Different state Medicaid rules and administration approaches continue to propagate inequities in health care access and outcomes. People of color or socioeconomically disadvantaged residents of various states suffer the most from that reality.

That's the truth.

The whole truth.

Nothing but the truth.

Key Stakeholder Reactions to Reform Efforts

"When plunder becomes a way of life for a group of men in a society, over the course of time, they create for themselves a legal system that authorizes it and a moral code that glorifies it." – Frederic Bastiat

Policy is a tool wielded by special interests to protect their market position and enhance their enterprise value. While patients, purchasers, payers, providers, and producers all had varied reactions to health reform efforts, they had in common the desire to come out ahead. Self-preservation.

Purchasers decided to shift more health care costs to consumers via higher deductibles and cost-sharing arrangements. A preferred alternative would have been a decision by purchasers to design and offer higher-value health benefits to consumers. Those higher-value health benefit plans would have been designed to deliver the best care and optimal health outcomes.

Higher deductibles are the favored approach by employers to shift health benefit costs to employees. Employers are the most aggressive purchaser employing this strategy. Manifesting this reality is the fact that the average employer-sponsored health plan deductible more than tripled in the decade since the enactment of the Affordable Care Act (ACA).

This strategy seemed to pay off for employers who were subsequently able to reduce the growth rate of health benefit premiums. Even though part of the ACA included creating individual insurance exchanges, more than 150 million people continued to access health plan benefits through their employer. At its peak, the ACA individual exchanges only enrolled approximately 20 million people. While the individual exchanges only enrolled about 20 million people, additional provisions in the ACA expanded coverage benefits via other means. Those additional provisions included new rules allowing dependents to stay on their parent's insurance till they were 26. Expansion of the Medicaid program also increased coverage benefits to millions more.

Given the current design and functioning of the American health care ecosystem, employers care about health care costs and health reform efforts. In several surveys of small to medium-sized businesses, health care costs, health care reform, and economic growth were the top three issues that had the most significant impact on their business decisions.

Looking at the situation slightly differently, the actions of the American health care cartel have the most significant impact on the business decisions of small to medium-sized businesses. Health care spending is the most potent drag on economic growth in America. The actions of the American health care cartel continue to drive health care spending higher, with no hope in sight.

As costs of higher deductibles started crippling the middle-class and squashing the poor, consumers reacted to higher deductibles by skipping preventive visits and other recommend health care encounters. Other consumers chose to remain uninsured, primarily due to affordability issues. They planned to delay seeking care until they qualified for Medicare or Medicaid coverage.

Several examples of low-income patients waiting with long lists of ailments flooded the airwaves pending the full implementation of the ACA and in the years since. According to surveys conducted by the CDC and the National Health Interview Survey (NHIS), 25-percent to 44-percent of the survey respondents indicated they were uninsured all or part of the two years from 2012 to 2013. Since they lacked insurance coverage, the survey respondents indicated that high costs prevented them from filling their prescription drugs in that time frame. There are several examples of this pattern of behavior leading to worsening of chronic illness and even death.

Declining rates of Americans who report having a primary care provider are also an emerging trend in response to health reform efforts. Partially explaining this emerging trend are primary care shortages in many health care markets. Other reasons like health care consumer attitudes towards preventive care have also been a known factor. Young adults and middle-aged Americans are the two groups in American society least likely to have a primary care physician or have a provider organization they routinely engage. Young adults typically feel invincible (at least I did when I was in my twenties) and don't engage the health care ecosystem for preventive care. Middle-age folks, on the other hand, may see a greater need for preventive care. Despite recognizing the need, responsibilities at home and work typically take up most of their time and limit opportunities for self-care or engaging a provider for preventive care services.

Most providers struggle to profit from value-based payment models. In the early days of the ACO program, most model participants did not achieve any savings. Some that earned savings failed to report quality metrics and didn't get awarded a bonus. Some that managed to reduce their spending didn't reduce it by a large enough margin to earn a shared savings bonus. The small cohort of ACOs who managed to achieve savings sufficiently significant enough to generate a shared savings bonus were rewarded with more challenging targets to meet the following year.

Given the self-defeating design of the ACO model, provider organizations, especially hospital-centric health systems, dropped out of the program after sustaining significant financial losses. Although CMS has attempted several iterations of the ACO model, retaining the self-defeating design of the ACO model construct will always be the ACO model's Achilles heel.

Some provider organizations also responded to health reform efforts by exploring various approaches to gaming risk-sharing arrangements. One standard method to gaming risk-sharing arrangements is selectively targeting patients for inclusion in specific risk-sharing arrangements. Some providers avoided enrolling highly complex patients with multiple chronic illnesses. Others avoided enrolling too many healthy patients. Others engaged in up-coding to exploit Risk Corridors (RC) and increase risk adjustment payments.

The different strategies employed were by design. Complex patients with multiple chronic illnesses usually have a long history of high health care spending. As a result, the provider organizations that sign them up can negotiate a higher benchmark payment from payers as they seek to generate shared savings. Some provider organizations seek to enroll less complex patients who don't have a long history of high health care spending. They pursue this approach with the hope that they can discover various ways to demand risk-adjusted payments for the patient lives they manage. Risk adjustments allow them to negotiate a higher benchmark payment than the managed population's historical health care spending would indicate.

Additional provider reactions to health reform have been decisions by many provider organizations to stop accepting new Medicare or Medicaid patients. Since many providers that have stopped taking Medicare and Medicaid patients are primary care providers, many Medicare and Medicaid patients have insurance coverage but minimal access to preventive care. As a result, those Medicare and Medicaid patients don't get the preventative care they need to optimize health outcomes. They often deteriorate at home while exasperatedly clutching their insurance coverage cards.

Adults with Medicaid are usually both poorer and sicker than low-income adults with commercial health insurance. Multiple chronic conditions, functional limitations, and mental health issues typically manifest within Medicaid patient populations. It didn't surprise anyone who knows the hustle that some provider organizations have decided to avoid Medicaid patients like the plague. With pressure to remain financially viable, providers responded to health reform efforts by increasing productivity volume. Squeezing additional patients into their daily schedule meant that some visits were scheduled for 10-to-15 minutes. As such, providers typically have limited time to attend to patients during a single visit.

Medicaid doesn't have the best record as a payer. In fact, in most American health care markets, Medicaid is usually the lowest reimbursing payer. A low reimbursing payer usually with the most extended Account Receivable (AR) days outstanding. In addition to the reasons mentioned above, other typical reasons for provider resistance to accepting Medicaid patients include the significant paperwork involved in registering as a Medicaid provider, reporting requirements, billing requirements, and practice capacity.

Some provider organizations like large dialysis providers have mostly stuck to old, nefarious ways of doing business instead of pursuing innovative care delivery and payment approaches. One of the most prominent and most notorious dialysis providers is DaVita Healthcare Partners (DaVita). According to Department of Justice (DOJ) press releases, in fiscal year 2015, DaVita agreed to pay 800 million dollars in fines to resolve claims that it violated the False Claims Act. DaVita was accused of paying kickbacks to induce the referral of patients to its dialysis clinics. DaVita was also accused of knowingly creating unnecessary waste and billing the federal government for it.

DaVita "allegedly" targeted certain physicians with lucrative opportunities to acquire and or sell an interest in DaVita dialysis clinics to which the provider's patients would be referred for treatment. Subsequently, DaVita prevented the physicians from referring their patients to other dialysis providers through non-compete and non-disparagement agreements with the physicians. The press release indicated that DaVita "allegedly" first used information gathered from numerous sources to identify physicians or physician groups with significant patient populations suffering from renal disease within a specific geographic area. DaVita "allegedly" would then gather detailed information about the physicians or physician group to determine if they would be a "winning practice." In one transaction, they labeled a physician group a "winning practice" because the physicians were "young and in debt."

In a second case from fiscal year 2015, DaVita "allegedly" directed its employees to maximize revenue by creating unnecessary waste and then billing the federal government for it. After a whistleblower notified the authorities and CMS eventually modified how it reimburses dialysis providers for administering the drugs in question, DaVita "allegedly" changed its operational guidance to its employees. They dramatically reduced their unnecessary waste once it became unprofitable to waste the drugs in question.

Like other members of the American health care cartel, DaVita is a dominant market force that is well-connected to other members of the American health care cartel. I don't want to single out DaVita since they aren't the only bad actors out there. I wanted to highlight what many consider eye-popping fines levied against the same company in the same fiscal year. DaVita continues to do business with state and federal governments despite many instances of documented wrongdoing and billions in fines paid over the years.

Since this type of activity is considered White-collar crime, it must not be that harmful. In reality, the types of crimes "allegedly" perpetrated by DaVita in the cases mentioned above are more dangerous than violent crimes. DaVita's "alleged" crimes destroyed the present and future of its victims. It undermined American prosperity. It undermined faith in the American health care ecosystem.

With more recent reform efforts like the Executive Order (EO) on Kidney Care signed by President Trump, DaVita, other dialysis providers, and affiliates in the American health care cartel remain poised to exploit loopholes. The mandatory End-Stage Renal Disease Treatment Choices (ETC) model included in the EO is intended to incentivize dialysis providers to deliver care in patients' homes. While the goal of home-based care is the right one, the model design has too many glaring loopholes. Loopholes that a crafty American health care cartel member like DaVita is quite adept at exploiting.

In fiscal year 2018, DOJ issued a press release indicating that it had recovered 2.8 billion dollars in fines from False Claims Act cases that year. The press release showed that recoveries in the 30-years since Congress substantially strengthened the civil False Claims Act totaled more than 59 billion dollars. While 2.8 billion dollars or 59 billion dollars is a lot of money in most scenarios, compared to the trillions of dollars sloshing around the American health care industry, it is barely a drop in the bucket. What is also clear is that most large corporations paying these "hefty" fines typically come out ahead.

No one usually goes to jail.

No one gets murdered by arresting police officers.

The 2018 DOJ press release also highlighted some producers. The most significant single recovery highlighted in the press release came from the drug and medical device industry.

AmerisourceBergen Corporation and certain of its subsidiaries paid 625 million dollars in fines for "allegedly" circumventing necessary safeguards intended to preserve the nation's drug supply integrity. They did so while profiting from the repackaging of certain drugs supplied to cancer-stricken patients.

Cancer.

American health care cartel members have no shame.

No limits. None.

The 2018 DOJ press release also highlighted misdeeds of pharmaceutical companies like United Therapeutics Corporation and Pfizer. United Therapeutics Corporation, a seller of pulmonary arterial hypertension (PAH) drugs, paid 210 million dollars in fines for "allegedly" using a foundation as an illegal conduit to pay the co-pay obligations of thousands of Medicare patients taking its PAH drugs. Pfizer "allegedly" used the same strategy and subsequently paid approximately 24 million dollars in fines. I guess United Therapeutics Corporation would be better off retaining the same caliber of esoteric knowledge experts—lawyers, accountants, and former regulators or legislators—that Pfizer has on-demand.

Not to be left out, payers also received an honorable mention in the same DOJ press release. The DOJ filed a series of complaints against UnitedHealth Group Inc. (UHG). DOJ "alleges" that UHG knowingly obtained inflated risk adjustment payments based on untruthful and inaccurate information about the health status of beneficiaries enrolled in UHG's Medicare Advantage Plans throughout the United States.

While the DOJ press release also highlighted False Claims Act violations by providers, I didn't think it was necessary to keep dragging the point out since I believe I've gotten my point across. And this chapter is getting too long.

American health care cartel members react to reform efforts in the same way.

They complain and obfuscate.

They identify new ways to exploit existing loopholes.

They create new loopholes.

If any loopholes manage to get closed with the implementation of new reforms, American health care cartel members influence the reform process to facilitate the creation of new loopholes. The loopholes included are by design. They enable American health care cartel members to continue to profit while American taxpayers suffer and American prosperity decays.

Unfortunately for American health care consumers and taxpayers, the American health care cartel's exploitation of loopholes obscures America's path to prosperity.

Loopholes persist because the American health care cartel retains its power over the American health care ecosystem.

The American health care cartel can only retain and wield its power because of campaign finance corruption, partisan gerrymandering, and voter suppression laws.

Campaign finance corruption, partisan gerrymandering, and voter suppression laws persist because American institutions were designed to uphold White supremacy.

American institutions weren't designed to establish an equitable, merit-based American democracy.

That's the truth.

The whole truth.

Nothing but the truth.

Uncompetitive Market Dynamics

"I swore never to be silent whenever and wherever human beings endure suffering and humiliation. We must take sides. Neutrality helps the oppressor, never the victim." – Elise Wiesel

Providers, especially physicians, have the market power to control prices for their services since they are the critical component of any care continuum. The essential nature of their involvement is mainly protected by licensure requirements associated with delivering most health care services. Since their role in the care continuum is protected, providers primarily responded to health reform efforts by increasing the pace of consolidation. As a result, most provider markets are highly consolidated.

In most local American health care markets, there are one to three dominant provider organizations that determine the prices and how much success health reform efforts will have in those markets. As such, the market dynamics that determine medical service prices and per capita health care costs continue to be worsened by harmful stakeholder consolidation.

Study after study continues to highlight the harmful effects of provider consolidation. Hospital consolidations usually raise prices without any improvement in quality or patient experience. As providers pursued a consolidation strategy to gain more market power, payers went on a similar consolidation mission. Consolidation is the preferred approach used by both stakeholder groups. With sufficient market power, payers or providers assume that the counterparty with weaker market power can't maintain a financially viable business in that health care market unless they come to terms with the counterparty with more substantial market power.

While the viewpoint mentioned above is theoretically accurate, some provider organizations, especially hospitals, refuse to negotiate even if they have weaker market power. Instead, those provider organizations focus on adopting a business strategy focused on charging patients and payers out-of-network rates for their services. Out-of-network rates are typically several multiples higher than the average negotiated reimbursement rate for the delivered health care services. Out-of-Network billing is the preferred go-to-market approach for hospitals with no proximate competition in their community. Those hospitals know that patients in crisis won't have any good alternatives and will eventually seek care at nearby out-of-network providers or risk deteriorating or dying on their prolonged journey to a distant in-network provider.

Early indication is that uncompetitive market dynamics will worsen in the aftermath of the COVID-19 pandemic. While there was some expectation that providers might be keen to embrace value-based payments in the aftermath of the COVID-19 pandemic, there's no sign that's the case. This expectation surfaced in the early days of the COVID-19 pandemic when providers using fully capitated models were financially sound while providers fully dedicated to fee-for-service revenues were hurting as the lockdowns went into effect and providers had to close their offices.

American health care cartel members seeking to profit from health reform are shaping the destination to their benefit, prolonging the duration of the shift to value-based payments, and adding new layers of cost for low-value activities. For example, EHR systems and medical device makers don't envision increased profitability by making their systems interoperable. As a result, they usually design their systems and devices to limit interoperability. The push for and against health care reform takes several forms. The most common approaches are campaign contributions, advertising, and lobbying.

Campaign contributions usually come from different sources and are delivered directly or indirectly to support or restrict health reform efforts. Sources of campaign contributions include individuals, corporations, and trade associations representing various special interest groups. While there were more stringent laws limiting amounts and sources of campaign contributions, the decision by the U.S. Supreme Court in 2010 opened the proverbial floodgates.

The 2010 Citizens United versus Federal Election Commission (FEC) decision by the U.S. Supreme Court classified political spending as a form of free speech protected under the First Amendment. Since free speech implies that speech should be unrestricted by law, political spending got to bask in the protection offered in the First Amendment and became unrestricted. With the U.S. Supreme Court's blessing, corporations and unions found it much easier to spend unlimited amounts to influence campaigns. New regulations also empowered them to hide the source of that spending.

The most cynical part of my mind would like to link the Citizens United decision to a coordinated backlash to the election of President Obama. However, I think America was already on the path to establishing a more corrupt campaign finance ecosystem. I think the U.S. Supreme Court would've likely ruled the same way even if Senator McCain won the 2008 election.

<u>All that aside, I'd like to embrace my conspiracy theorist mindset for a minute.</u>

My conspiracy theory is that American oligarchs—clandestine association of the wealthiest White males who actually run America—were frightened when President Obama, a Black man, won the 2008 election. They activated their minions on the U.S. Supreme Court to play their part in the onslaught against American voters who dared to elect a Black man as president.

Their minions on the U.S. Supreme Court legalized obscene amounts of corrupt financial influence to poison the already compromised American campaign finance ecosystem.

Oligarchs control most of the wealth in America and weren't banking on President Obama winning the 2008 election. With President Obama's win, they felt like they were losing their stranglehold on America.

The inherent fear American oligarchs have is rooted in a sinking feeling that <u>We the People</u> were finally coming to our senses. They believe we will eventually come after them with proverbial (or actual) "torches" and "pitchforks." Guilty conscience.

The 2010 mid-term elections were the most heavily financed mid-term elections up to that point in American history. Democrats got swept out in large numbers. That election cycle legitimized the Tea Party (birther) movement and elevated their ruling minions. The rest, as they say, is history.

The American oligarchs played it masterfully because the narrative most mass media outlets went with was that lower-income, low-skilled White people were pushed to the brink when President Obama was elected.

We are supposed to believe that they subsequently organized a political machine that would go on to reconstitute state and national legislatures in the ensuing decade.

In reality, America's oligarchs were behind all of it. The masses got played, as usual.

The only group that has consistently profited from the Citizens United decision are American oligarchs.

The American masses that fell for it are mostly still stuck.

Living in squalor.

Unable to make ends meet.

Blindly capitulating to the whims of ruling minions controlled by American oligarchs.

<u>Ok. I've gotten that out of my system for now.</u>

Campaign contributions are used to elect legislators and appoint public officials that are subsequently beholden to or aligned with the interests of the American health care cartel. With the large war chests that cartel-sponsored legislators can accumulate, those that oppose the American health care cartel usually don't have a leg to stand on. The billions of dollars American health care cartel members invest in "campaign contributions" each election cycle doesn't just come with strings attached. Those investment dollars come with veto power. Veto power capable of ensuring that paradigm-shifting health reform proposals are always Dead On Arrival (DOA).

Minimizing competition is the only "winning" strategy the American health care cartel can conjure. Mediocre. Unimaginative. Lazy. Lethal.

Every cartel-sponsored legislator is evaluated to ensure they aren't interested in using the powers of the government to promote competition in health care markets. In rare instances, some legislators start beating the drums of government interventions that encourage market competition. The American health care cartel is quick to deploy additional capital to "educate" legislators on how to think and vote on any potential paradigm-shifting health reform proposals. Some legislators only beat those drums to shake more money out of the American health care cartel. It is just a ruse, a shakedown. Mediocre. Unimaginative. Lazy. Lethal.

America refers to the process of "educating" legislators as "lobbying." In countries that know what the deal is, paying "facilitators" to "educate" legislators on ways of thinking and voting is referred to as <u>bribery</u>.

The American health care lobby is one of the most prolific and formidable lobbies in the game. Some of the most prolific health care lobbying groups are also card-carrying members of the American health care cartel.

The Pharmaceutical Research and Manufacturers of America (PhRMA), American Medical Association (AMA), American Hospital Association (AHA), and America's Health Insurance Plans (AHIP) are formidable lobbying groups. They fiercely defend their respective industry groups' desire to continue to extract economic rents from the American health care ecosystem.

According to the website www.opensecrets.org, in 2008, when the Affordable Care Act (ACA) was being negotiated, more than 3,500 people were registered as health care lobbyists. That's 35 lobbyists for every Senator and more than six lobbyists for every Representative.

In 2008 and 2009, more than one billion dollars was deployed by health care lobbyists. That's a lot of "education."

With the election of President Trump in 2016, the health care lobby scaled its spending to higher heights. Health care lobbying consistently eclipsed 500 million dollars every year President Trump was in office. The spending peaked at 622 million dollars in 2020.

According to the website www.opensecrets.org, in 2020, lobbyists representing pharmaceutical and health product stakeholders spent more than 300 million dollars "educating" legislators. Hospitals and nursing homes spent more than 110 million dollars on similar efforts.

Their investments paid off as billions of taxpayer-funded stimulus dollars were directed to pharmaceutical companies, hospitals, and nursing homes in return. As the COVID-19 pandemic raged on and American health care cartel members padded their balance sheets with stimulus funds, thousands of primarily Black and Brown people were deteriorating or dying in their homes.

Deteriorating or dying with limited access to care.

While lobbying is designed to "educate" legislators, advertising is how the American health care cartel brainwashes the masses.

Advertising is where mass media outlets in the American health care cartel do their best work. It's an art form at this point. American health care consumers can easily recognize clearly labeled advertisements and campaign commercials for what they are. They aren't too attuned to American health care cartel propaganda hardwired into the entertainment content they consume.

From television shows like ER that captured the nation's imagination to every implausible iteration spurned ever since American health care cartel propaganda continues to infiltrate the subconscious of the masses. Hospital-centric acute care isn't the foundation for any effectively designed health care ecosystem. If made for television propaganda is believed, technological improvements to the current health care ecosystem and enhanced hospital care are what we need most: that and some stunning medical personnel.

Media outlets and platforms capitulate to the demands of the American health care cartel. Like everyone else, they also like income they can extract from the bloated American health care ecosystem. As they laugh all the way to the bank, the masses they should be illuminating and activating with the truth are being fed half-truths and whole lies.

Those half-truths and whole lies continue to obscure America's path to prosperity.

In an ideal scenario, media outlets and platforms would have evolved their business models to sustainably fulfill their appropriate role in a civilized society.

They are supposed to <u>highlight the root causes of societal ills while holding accountable the institutions</u> that inflict harm on the masses.

Instead, most media outlets and platforms seem to be settling into their role as propaganda machines for the American health care cartel.

By pulling levers of campaign contributions, lobbying, and advertising, the American health care cartel maintains its stranglehold on America's path to prosperity. Campaign finance corruption, partisan gerrymandering, and voter suppression laws embolden the American health care cartel in its quest to subjugate America.

Emboldened American health care cartel members act with impunity and keep most American health care markets consolidated and thus beholden to the whims of the American health care cartel. While most American health care markets are beholden to the whims of the American health care cartel, the needs of American health care consumers and taxpayers are routinely ignored.

Competition drives performance excellence.

Uncompetitive market dynamics curtail the utility of operating in capitalistic markets.

Uncompetitive markets embrace bureaucracy and stifle paradigm-shifting innovation.

Uncompetitive markets must be dismantled.

Uncompetitive market dynamics broadly benefit the American health care cartel. However, provider members of the cartel extract the most significant benefits from uncompetitive health care markets.

Unfortunately for health care consumers, as provider organizations benefit from operating in uncompetitive health care markets, patients are stuck in markets with fewer choices and higher prices. There is enough blame to go around, though.

Insurance should aim to be more than legalized extortion.

For most consumers, the experience is just paying what you're told to pay.

Praying that you never have to use it.

And when you do need to use it, claims processing is usually a hassle.

It's all the same, car, life, homeowners, health, etcetera.

That's the truth.

The whole truth.

Nothing but the truth.

Non-adherence to Evidence-based Clinical Guidelines

"Almost all quality improvement comes via simplification of design, processes, and procedures." — Tom Peters

It routinely takes the clinical practice guidelines lifecycle almost 20-years before leading evidence-based practices are adopted as the standard-of-care across the American health care ecosystem.

The clinical practice guidelines process usually originates in the research domain. From the research domain, clinical practice guidelines transition to the policy domain. From the policy domain, it transitions to the organizational or managerial domain. From the organizational or managerial domain, it transitions to the societal domain.

Process transitions aren't always smooth or timely. The clinical practice guidelines process can also originate from evaluation studies conducted in the societal, organizational, or managerial domain. Outcomes of the evaluation studies often inform the establishment of research priorities and other activities within the research domain.

The research domain is focused on knowledge synthesis. By evaluating scientific evidence on problems, interventions, and implementations, principal investigators and organizations supporting the process at this stage conduct systematic reviews of evidence that has been validated locally and globally. As the process transitions from research to policy, additional activities are pursued in the research domain.

Efforts to set priorities and anticipate winning policy strategies often translate to creating knowledge summaries to facilitate discussions with policymakers.

The additional step of creating a knowledge summary is often necessary because policymakers aren't fond of reading lengthy research reports. Most people aren't. Just saying.

The development of knowledge summaries wouldn't be complete without a comprehensive understanding of health systems. Through the research effort and validation of evidence, it is essential to ascertain that one compares apples to apples. Information on the health systems contributing to the body of proof should be validated and critical success factors identified.

Ideally, health systems information should be validated across the following factors: leadership or governance, service delivery model, workforce health, information technology, and medical interventions.

Successfully navigating the policy domain requires an in-depth knowledge of the rules of the game. The game at this stage is mostly about exchanging knowledge, appropriately filtering that knowledge to connect with influential audiences, and amplifying as needed to reach the broadest audience.

Guidance assets are also required to advance efforts at this stage of the game. One of the most impactful guidance assets is personal experiences. Personal experiences are refined into powerful stories that are shared to connect with audiences on a human level.

Additional guidance assets include political judgment, interest groups, policy legacies, societal values, external events, colloquial evidence, and other sector resources.

Advancing beyond the policy domain usually involves a contentious transition to the organizational or managerial environment. Often, the feedback loop that facilitates this transition starts with matching desired health outcomes to population health needs. Once population health needs are prioritized, policy proposals undertake an iterative process to establish the standard of care in service delivery. An iterative process heavily influenced by the American health care cartel. The influence ensures they are positioned to benefit from the adoption of the updated standard of care.

Transitions from the policy domain to service delivery can be very challenging. Challenges arise because standards of care originating from the policy domain aren't always welcomed by the organizations and people required to adopt them.

The societal domain almost runs concurrently as members of society are usually involved in related testing and implementation planning efforts. The desired outcomes that drive folks at the intersection of organizational and societal domains are improved health and equity, improved efficiency, and risk protection.

In addition to transition gaps that occur as clinical practice guidelines advance between domains, delayed adoption also occurs because of health data fragmentation and the American health care ecosystem's cultural bias against disruptive health care innovation.

This unfortunate reality leaves millions of patients following substandard care paths. Those substandard care paths could have been avoided if the American health care ecosystem was enabled with higher-value information technology infrastructure.

In addition to transition delays, technical gaps, and cultural bias against disruptive health care innovation, the shortage of higher-value health care workers in many states continues to limit the adoption of leading evidence-based clinical delivery.

To reduce the burden on physicians and effectively support patient care needs, several non-physician members of the clinical care team can execute leading evidence-based clinical guidelines. While non-physician members of the clinical care team are licensed to practice with a relatively broad scope of practice, state regulations often restrict the scope of practice of non-physicians.

Nurse Practitioners (NPs) and Physician Assistants (PAs) are the most impacted by those restrictions. Beyond NPs and PAs, Registered Nurses (RNs) and other licensed members of the clinical care team are also adversely affected by the arbitrary state-level rules on scope of practice.

Beyond the inefficiencies propagated by scope of practice limitations, not practicing at the top of their license can be frustrating and stressful for most licensed professionals. Self-actualization is vital to emotional well-being. Consistently being restricted to operating below one's capability, training or licensure can be mentally stressful and even debilitating.

Many non-physician members of the clinical care team have formed trade associations and lobby for expanded scope of practice authorities in different states. Unfortunately for them, the American health care cartel deploys more lobbyists to counteract their efforts. Most states have some restrictions on the scope of practice of licensed professionals like NPs or PAs.

The most restrictive states mandate supervision, delegation, or team management of NPs by physicians. Those restrictions are arbitrary and often unnecessary since NPs can accurately evaluate patients, diagnose, order, interpret orders and diagnostic tests, and initiate and manage treatments, including prescribing medication and managing adherence.

Liberal strongholds like California and Massachusetts and Conservative strongholds like Texas and Tennessee have historically enforced stringent scope of practice restrictions on NPs. This fact highlights the reality that the American health care cartel has activated both sides of the aisle to implement scope of practice rules.

Scope of practice restrictions impedes the ability of care teams and health systems to adopt leading evidence-based clinical guidelines. In addition to not adhering to leading evidence-based clinical guidelines, utilizing NPs and PAs below their scope of practice is an expensive proposition. A costly proposition designed to enrich members of the American health care cartel. As the American health care cartel laughs all the way to the bank, care team members practicing below NPs and PAs have some of their most advanced work taken over by NPs and PAs. NPs and PAs who aren't allowed to practice at the top of their license. As the saying goes, crap rolls downhill.

Evidence-based clinical guidelines development, evaluation, and translation to different care settings are uncoordinated and complex. According to the Institute of Medicine (IOM), guidelines are systematically developed statements to assist practitioner and patient decisions about appropriate health care for specific clinical circumstances.

Several critical components enable clinical guidelines to lead to clinical recommendations. Factors such as patient values, acceptability, the rigor of evidence, costs, and benefits versus harms, help determine what clinical recommendations are shared with the patient and ultimately what care path and standard of care the patient is advised to follow.

There are several organizations and entities involved in the clinical practice guidelines lifecycle. Each entity works within its prescribed domain and also across fields. Most of the organizations and entities involved in the clinical practice guidelines lifecycle are quality measurement industrial complex members.

The quality measurement industrial complex is the stronghold of the most prolific and low-value esoteric knowledge experts exploiting the bloated American health care ecosystem.

They thrive on complexity and pursue low-value activities due to the innate unimportance of the quality measurement industrial complex in the grand scheme of things.

Often partnering up with the conference industrial complex (they also have trade associations), quality measurement industrial complex members are keen to meet up at glitzy health care conferences to collectively admire the complexity of the American health care ecosystem. Complexity they thrive on. The complexity serves as the primary, or only, justification for their professional existence. They often ascend to stages reminiscent of concert venues and wax poetic in contrived terms about the many reasons why quality measurement activities aren't delivering value across the American health care ecosystem.

The conference industrial complex is keen to partner with the quality measurement industrial complex because many conference event spaces were designed and built for American health care industry gatherings. COVID-19 devastated the utilization of conference event space. I assume members of the conference industrial complex and members of the quality measurement industrial complex are likely collaborating on ways to cram as many souls back into conference event spaces as soon COVID-19 restrictions are lifted.

The prevalent business model in the conference event industry is a model that generates rental fees from event room usage and ancillary services like catering, furniture rental, etcetera. This business model doesn't encourage the conference industrial complex members to promote innovation that disrupts current business models that generate revenue from in-person meetings. Yes. Airlines, hotels, municipalities' etcetera are in on this hustle as well.

The quality measurement industrial complex, on the other hand, is incentivized to prolong the clinical practice guidelines lifecycle.

With armies of review panels and months of discourse and debates, a systematic review of evidence is manually completed in a highly fragmented and disconnected fashion. The lack of information sharing is so pervasive that sometimes two different researchers affiliated with the same academic institution can be working on identical or similar clinical practice guidelines without collaborating with each other.

Technology solutions like a centralized, national or global database of all clinical practice guidelines could be created. Unfortunately, efforts to advance technology to improve the efficacy of the clinical practice guidelines lifecycle have been met with stiff resistance from members of the quality measurement industrial complex. Like much opposition to technology-enabled change writ large, resistance in this context also comes down to protecting incumbents and existing jobs. This mentality is also broadly applicable to the clinical trials lifecycle.

One of the more irritating things about the current business model embraced by the quality measurement industrial complex is that it remains wasteful and promotes unnecessary delays in the clinical practice guidelines lifecycle. When evaluating challenges at the intersection of quality measurement and health reform, the situation usually worsens.

Improving quality, cost, and health are the central goals of the Triple Aim and the value-based care movement. Challenges arise while trying to get all stakeholders and interested parties to reach a consensus on measuring the elements of the Triple Aim. While reaching an agreement was practically impossible, some of the compromises struck didn't yield beneficial results either.

For example, with the value-based care models being tested by the CMS Innovation Center (CMMI), model participants were asked in many cases to indicate which quality measures they wanted to report on. Like clockwork, the American health care cartel jumped to action and used the flexibilities offered to introduce a slew of different quality measurements. Flexibilities meant that participating providers could choose the quality measures they wanted to report on. Measures they could excel on.

As different providers were being evaluated using various measures, it became abundantly clear that it would be complicated and almost impossible to compare multiple providers' performance in the same model.

Further complicating the situation were providers who failed to report any quality metrics and others whose reported metrics had been compromised.

The preferred business model of the quality measurement industrial complex generates more revenues with complex clinical practices, lengthy guidelines lifecycles, convoluted processes, increased volume, and overall complexity.

That's the truth.

The whole truth.

Nothing but the truth.

Potential Solutions

"If the solution is not affordable and accessible, it is not a solution."
– Dr. Devi Shetty

Creating a new product is only one way to innovate. On its own, it provides the lowest return on investment and the least competitive advantage. The Ten Types of Innovation Framework developed by partners at the Doblin Group, a management consulting firm, evaluates various ways to identify new opportunities beyond products and develop viable innovations. While a published book of the same name manages to explain ten different types of innovation models, it doesn't account for the power of an institution like the American health care cartel to influence the viability of any innovation.

The Ten Types of Innovation Framework pursues innovation across three channel strategies. First, it explores tactics aimed at changing configurations. Second, it explores tactics aimed at changing offerings. Finally, it explores tactics aimed at changing experiences.

Tactics designed to innovate via configurations include innovating the approach organizations profit, innovating the alignment of talent and assets, innovating the nature of network partnerships to create value, and innovating the process by which work is completed.

Tactics designed to innovate via offerings include innovating a product's distinguishing features and functionality and innovating a product system's complementary products and services.

Tactics designed to innovate via experiences include innovating the enhancements that support service offerings, innovating how offerings are delivered to customers and users, innovating representation of offerings, and innovating the distinctive interactions with customers.

The Ten Types of Innovation Framework is as good as any other innovation framework to assess opportunities to improve American health care delivery and payments. The three questions that come to mind when I think about the Ten Types of Innovation Framework in the context of American health care are: How can we reinvent or recombine solutions to deliver unique value? How do we engage customers differently to provide value? And, how do we fundamentally alter the way we capture value?

Disruptive innovation is most effective when transformation efforts are focused on meeting user needs, not incrementally improving the existing system. In 2007, Taxicab Magic (acquired by Verifone in 2015, spun out as Curb Mobility in 2018) invented electronic ground travel booking and payment on mobile phones. It created a mobile app connecting people to safe, reliable rides from professional taxis and other-for-hire drivers in cities nationwide. In 2009, UberCab was founded by Garrett Camp and Travis Kalanik. They officially launched Uber's services and mobile app in 2011. Uber epitomizes disruption. The company has fundamentally changed the way we think about grabbing a ride. They created a brand new experience for consumers and differentiated opportunities for producers.

While I'm well aware of the many controversies surrounding Uber's business model and toxic corporate culture, the fact remains that the world is no longer bound to the antiquated manner in which users solicited rides from for-hire drivers. I'm incredibly grateful as a Black man who could never seem to get an empty cab to stop as I frantically waved and watched them drive past me to pick up someone else. That scenario played out a couple of times I visited New York City pre-Uber. Yes, the other person I was shunned for was always a White person.

Beyond service delivery improvements, Uber's growth also decimated the bloated market value of a New York City (NYC) Taxi Cab License. The NYC Taxi Cab License went from peak values of over one million dollars in 2014 to less than 150 thousand dollars in 2019. The main losers were the NYC institutions who extorted exorbitant fees for the Taxi Cab licenses they issued and the Taxi Cab drivers who took out loans to pay for NYC Taxi Cab licenses at peak prices. The main winners were users who embraced a simpler, affordable, and equitable (most of the time) ecosystem. Uber's founders, investors, and employees also did very well for themselves

Despite the significant time and resource commitment to health reform, progress is slow and considerable opportunities exist to catalyze lasting, systemic change.

We must spend smarter on behalf of the American people by scaling what works and stopping what doesn't.

Problem 1. Technical, policy, political, and market barriers obstruct critical pathways to system-wide adoption of effective value-based payments.

Problem 2. Key stakeholders avoid being accountable for complex populations, while many just shift costs to others.

Problem 3. Dominant groups create market dynamics that limit the value realized from payment reform efforts.

Problem 4. Even when incentives are aligned, some entrenched barriers to system-wide adherence to evidence-based clinical guidelines persist.

Objective. Create a higher-value American health care ecosystem that efficiently delivers the best care and optimal health.

<u>Strategy</u>. Change system incentives and promote leading practices.

Since the payment method determines who gets savings from waste reduction, we must focus on enabling payment methods and market dynamics that reward higher-value care delivery. If we change incentives, American health system stakeholders are likely to embrace cost-effective solutions that enable higher-value care delivery and improve population health outcomes. Opportunities exist to facilitate adoption when changing incentives alone are insufficient to allow system-wide adherence to leading evidence-based clinical practices.

<u>Tactic 1</u>. Accelerate the transition from fee-for-service to value-based payments.

To change system incentives, we must accelerate the transition to value-based payment methods by removing barriers to adoption and enhancing proven stakeholder solutions. Efforts to transition to value-based payments are slow and obstructed by significant obstacles. Thus, many value-based payment arrangements being tested or adopted have little or no financial risk and are still reliant on fee-for-service transaction infrastructure.

It is of great importance that significant public and private resources currently dedicated to advancing health reform aren't wasted. Thus, positioning critical efforts for maximum impact is a high-leverage approach to achieving systemic change. Pursuing value-enhancing system reforms not comprehensively addressed by ongoing efforts would ensure that future efforts focus on the highest-value reforms. Making the economic argument for value-based practices and promoting adoption requires partnerships with critical stakeholders to scale high-value solutions. Such alliances also create opportunities to actively challenge non-value enhancing regulations.

Potential actions to implement this tactic include: (1) Developing and evaluating sustainable business cases that promote solutions that work. (2) Rigorously evaluating the effectiveness of value-based payment models that include fee-for-service transaction architecture. (3) Piloting and evaluating health reform models that are not comprehensively addressed by ongoing or planned efforts. (4) Scaling models that improve treatment quality and health outcomes of complex populations. (5) Activating key stakeholders to demand more effective payment reform to reduce the cost of higher-value benefit designs. (6) Promoting higher-value health benefit design and the adoption of value-purchasing practices.

Tactic 2. Disrupt uncompetitive market dynamics

To enable higher-value care delivery across the entire American health care ecosystem, we must disrupt uncompetitive markets that resist reform and cause prices to rise. Most health care markets are highly concentrated and controlled by large health systems that have no viable business case to adopt value-based payments that shift care away from expensive hospital-based settings. The hospitals in these various health systems have significant fixed costs funded by the structure and financing of the current health system.

Costs are on the rise as market dynamics worsen. The surge is fueled by providers' desire to sustain revenues and profit. Acquiring significant market share and negotiation leverage allows providers to demand higher fees from payers and patients who have no viable local alternatives to turn to.

Potential actions to implement this tactic include: (1) Supporting legal challenges and policy-based efforts to reduce harmful stakeholder consolidation. (2) Promoting competition across stateliness by directing appropriate types and levels of care to centers of excellence. (3) Scaling reference pricing approaches that challenge cost structure and prices in similar markets.

<u>Tactic 3</u>. Challenge barriers to system-wide adherence to evidence-based clinical guidelines.

When changing incentives alone are insufficient, we must challenge entrenched barriers to health reform by promoting leading practices that enable higher-value care delivery. Even when incentives are aligned as they are within integrated health systems like Kaiser Permanente, which encompasses both payers and providers, the delivery of high-value care isn't always assured.

In 2015, Kaiser Permanente's 2,600 psychologists, therapists, and social workers staged a walkout to demand that Kaiser Permanente offer timely, quality mental health care at its psychiatry departments and clinics. The striking workers cited cases where some patients had to wait up to two months for follow-up appointments, prolonging the recovery process.

The system-wide dissemination of high-value, evidence-based care is also limited by persistent structural and cultural barriers that extend the gap between when evidence is created and clinical practice is updated.

Expensive labor and regulatory compliance are significant drivers of cost in the American health care ecosystem. Even when high-value workers possess the requisite experience to perform specific clinical tasks according to evidence-based guidelines, several realities stand in their way. Licensing requirements, health system policies, and government regulations limit their scope of practice while driving up the cost of employing or engaging authorized personnel.

Physicians are the authorized personnel for advanced clinical practice and are positioned as the most critical personnel to the viability of any health system. Physicians remain resistant to their loss of autonomy in clinical practice even though most have given up their independent practice.

Physicians can enable non-compliance in other clinical workers if they disagree with leading clinical practices guidelines.

To effectively promote evidence-based leading practices, we must focus on challenging structural and cultural barriers to system-wide adherence to evidence-based care delivery.

Potential actions to implement this tactic are both structural and cultural in nature. They include: (1) Increasing the supply of high-value health care workers that have been trained to adhere to evidence-based guidelines. (2) Enabling the adoption of value-based quality and outcomes measurement tools. (3) Reforming policies that inappropriately limit the scope of practice of health workers. (4) Developing effective change management messaging and dissemination tools. (5) Promoting collaboration among developers and disseminators of evidence-based clinical guidelines.

Advancing a health system reform agenda focused on changing incentives and promoting leading practices can transform the system if sustainable solutions are scaled effectively. Unfortunately for health care consumers, the American health care cartel exists and wields its power over the political industrial complex to undermine any reform efforts its members don't endorse.

The American health care cartel doesn't like any reforms that threaten its ability to extract economic rents from the complex, expensive, and inequitable American health care ecosystem.

When presented with health reform proposals, I would advise policymakers and members of the public to clarify four things:

1. Theory of change.

2. Validating evidence.

3. How the implementation of the proposed reforms will bend the cost curve.

4. How the American health care cartel will respond.

If the proposer's responses to those four questions don't pass the horse manure test, tell them to shop their snake oil elsewhere. Unfortunately, the political industrial complex and dominant market forces make my proposed solutions infeasible. While I would like to walk through the different ways the American health care cartel would undermine the strategy and tactics I mention above, I'm wary of turning this chapter into a never-ending epistle—a rather depressing one.

However, I will highlight some tactics the American health care cartel will likely use to undermine others' solutions. I will focus on reform pursued by the Trump Administration, proposals by the Biden-Sanders Unity task force health policy team, and recommendations by health reform experts listed on the 1% Steps for Health Care Reform Project website.

The Trump Administration made a lot of health reform promises. Most of those promises failed to materialize into enacted legislation. Attempts were made to use Executive Orders to reform health care. While Executive Orders can be helpful, they aren't permanent and are often subject to legal challenges.

Repealing and replacing the ACA was the stated health reform priority of the Trump Administration. Fortunately for health care consumers, even with a Republican majority in both chambers and President Trump in the White House, they couldn't figure out how to repeal and replace the ACA.

Although they weren't able to repeal and replace the ACA, they continued their relentless efforts to undermine and sabotage the ACA. In December 2017, Republicans in Congress passed, and President Trump signed the Tax Cuts and Jobs Act, eliminating the penalty for the ACA's individual mandate.

The Trump Administration got a price transparency rule across the finish line. Price transparency is essential to establishing competitive health care markets. Unfortunately, the American health care cartel was involved in the process. Their involvement ensured that the final price transparency rule didn't have any real shot at achieving its stated objective.

Some of the complicating factors were structural in nature. For example, the penalties for non-compliance were only a couple hundred dollars per day. Also, organizations weren't given a specific format or central repository to upload the data. Finally, forcing stakeholders to reveal prices will likely lead to a mean reversion or higher overall prices. Those who priced their services too low will raise their prices. Those who priced their services too high will likely focus on convincing others to increase their prices or dust off the consolidation playbook and acquire lower-cost competition.

Barely a few months after the final rule was published, the price transparency effort started to fall apart. The American health care cartel ensured that the regulatory agency (CMS) didn't have adequate resources for effective monitoring and oversight. Provider members of the American health care cartel complained about the exorbitant cost and labor hours they claim would be associated with reporting price data. It would appear that regulators are capitulating to the demands of the American health care cartel. In April 2021, CMS released its proposal to increase reimbursement for hospitals by 2.5 billion dollars while repealing part of the price transparency rule related to Medicare Advantage (MA) plans. I could write a whole book on MA plans. Those folks aren't messing around. At all.

In January 2021, the New England Journal of Medicine (NEJM) published an opinion editorial by Brad Smith, the outgoing Director of the CMS Innovation Center (CMMI). In the publication, Brad indicated that the vast majority of CMMI's models have not saved money. He also highlighted the fact that several models were on pace to lose billions of dollars. Similarly, he mentioned that majority of the models didn't show significant improvements in quality.

There are many reasons why CMMI, its expanded authorities, and its billion-dollar annual budget have failed to deliver savings or improve quality. The primary reason is that members of the American health care cartel continue to set CMMI's priorities. It's also not clear what CMMI's strategy is. I suspect that flaw is by design.

CMMI has pursued dozens of tactics repeatedly without first defining an overarching strategy or an integrated approach to creating a paradigm-shift. While I'm a tad critical of CMMI's impact, CMMI helped highlight the fact that there aren't any paths to sustainably adopting value-enhancing Alternative Payment Models (APMs) on fee-for-service transaction architecture.

The well-publicized drug price reduction efforts the Trump Administration pursued didn't amount to much. The changes related to drug prices that members of the Trump Administration implemented actually increased the prices of certain drugs.

CMMI announced the Direct Contracting (DC) Model. The DC Model is a population-based payment model that is designed to encourage competition by positioning new entrants for success. New entrant Direct Contracting Entities (DCEs) are permitted to start with as few as 250 beneficiaries.

Unfortunately for health care consumers, the American health care cartel rose up against the DC Model. Regulators eventually capitulated. In March 2021, CMMI announced it was indefinitely pausing the rollout of the most compelling DC Model, the DC Geo Model. Although DC model options like the professional and global were allowed to continue, regulators stopped accepting applications for new participants. Effectively condemning the DC Model to "circling the drain" status.

The DC Geo Model is especially compelling because, as configured, in addition to voluntary beneficiary alignment, automatic assignment of managed lives to participating DCEs is an option. By assigning lives to DCEs participating in the DC Geo Model, those DCEs would be empowered to redirect what they would have otherwise spent on marketing and beneficiary acquisition towards care delivery or additional savings. Marketing and beneficiary acquisition costs aren't trivial amounts. Advertisements promoting Medicare Advantage plans aren't cheap. Broadway Joe's teeth aren't going to pay for themselves. Not knocking his hustle. Just injecting some pop culture into the discourse.

The DC Geo Model was configured with sufficient flexibility for participating DCEs to reimagine the health care technology and services stack at scale. A reimagined technology and services stack that didn't have to be reliant on fee-for-service transaction architecture. A reimagined technology and services stack that didn't have to be hospital-centric.

Finally, DCEs participating in the DC Geo Model were required to establish patient care oversight boards. Oversight boards that would have ultimately given patients a seat and a voice at the decision-making table.

Although DC models weren't automatically destined to be the health reform panacea we've been waiting for, they were the boldest attempt at paradigm-shifting change to come out of CMMI since its inception.

Unfortunately for health care consumers, the ACO gang, and their allies, weren't fans. While ACOs continue to lose members and participants, their trade association saw the launch of the DC model as a potential death nail. A death nail that would render the ACO trade association worthless.

Changing the antecedent before ACO (Pioneer, Next Generation etcetera) does little to change the fact that the ACO model as configured is self-defeating and designed to achieve mediocre outcomes at best. ACOs are fundamentally flawed by design and destined for mediocrity. It's a shame that most health reform efforts continue to pivot back to iterations of a self-defeating model. The American health care cartel wins again.

Health reform efforts often fail to address many loopholes. That unfortunate reality reflects the overpowering influence of the American health care cartel. As such, paradigm-shifting opportunities to test new models of care and payment remain off-limits to CMMI.

Health care policy recommendations from the Biden-Sanders unity task force were similarly constrained. While much of it read like a laundry list of wishes the American health care cartel would never grant, some recommendations were basically handouts to the American health care cartel. Handouts that weren't designed to make American health care simple, affordable, and equitable.

The Biden-Sanders unity task force health care policy team was co-chaired by Rep. Pramila Jayapal and Vivek Murthy. Other members included: Donald Berwick, Abdul El-Sayed, Sherry Glied, Mary Kay Henry, Chris Jennings, and Rep. Robin Kelly. I've had the opportunity to speak with some of them. I consider all the task force members informed and respectable. Yet, I'm not sure what their strategy for paradigm-shifting change is. I also have no idea how they plan to bend the cost curve.

Merely allocating more capital to the American health care ecosystem doesn't address the root cause of cancer metastasizing at the intersection of White supremacy and American health care.

Proposed Solution 1: Reinvest in Public Health

Tactics and Key Activities

"Protect federal scientists from political influence, establish a comprehensive, national public health surveillance program for COVID-19 and future infectious diseases, recruit 100,000 contract tracers to help state and local health departments identify people at risk of contracting or spreading the coronavirus."

Complicating Factors. Reads very much like a jobs program and a handout to the states. Not sure why proposed solutions aren't simply designed to accomplish the stated objective efficiently. Recruiting 100,000 contact tracers, shoring up state and local budgets to fund the bloated American health care system without demanding fundamental reform. In addition, supporting the World Health Organization (WHO) doesn't strategically or meaningfully address the public health infrastructure deficit pervasive across states and municipalities across America.

Likely Outcomes. If the Democrats have the votes to pass legislation, they'll probably stick this proposal in a COVID-19 stimulus bill. Any appropriation received will be spent on addressing the current crisis. More money will be needed to support the crumbling public health infrastructure in the future. Finally, even if a magic wand is waved and all the tactics are magically implemented, the American health care cartel will remain intact. And the American health care ecosystem will remain complex, expensive, and inequitable.

Proposed Solution 2: Secure Universal Health Care through a Public Option

Tactics and Key Activities

"Give all Americans a choice to select a high-quality, affordable public option through the ACA marketplace. Administer the Public Option with the traditional Medicare program and exclude private payers. Cover all primary care

> with no co-payments. Negotiate prices with doctors and hospitals. Automatically enroll low-income Americans who don't qualify for Medicaid. Expand funding for ACA outreach and enrollment programs. Lower the Medicare enrollment age to 60. Empower states to use ACA innovation waivers and pursue statewide universal health care approaches. Increase investments in community health centers and rural health clinics with multi-year funding cycles. Expand National Health Services Corps."

<u>Complicating Factors</u>. Though ambitious, this proposal is Dead on Arrival (DOA). For several reasons. First, it hurts too many members of the American health care cartel. Providers and payers will fight it with every fiber of their being. Large employers will hate losing some of the leverage they have over their employees. Producers will likely support it since it opens up their pool of insured customers. In my experience, if providers, payers, and large employers are aligned against a reform effort, that effort isn't going anywhere. Second, the Public Option as configured isn't designed to solve the main fundamental issues plaguing the American health care ecosystem. The public option essentially seeks to expand insurance coverage.

<u>Likely Outcomes</u>. I don't think the Democrats will find the votes to pass Public Option legislation. They may not even bother if the Congressional Budget Office (CBO) or CMS Actuary forecasts an exorbitant implementation price tag. Finally, even if a magic wand is waved and all the tactics are magically implemented, the American health care cartel will remain intact. And the American health care ecosystem will remain complex, expensive, and inequitable.

Proposed Solution 3: Bring Down Drug Prices and Take on the Pharmaceutical Industry

<u>Tactics and Key Activities</u>
> "Take aggressive action to ensure that Americans do not pay more for prescription drugs than people in other advanced

economies. Empower Medicare to negotiate prescription drug prices for all public and private purchasers. Ensure and enforce that the price of brand-name and outlier generic drugs doesn't rise faster than the rate of inflation. Cap out-of-pocket drug costs for seniors. Ensure that effective treatments for chronic health conditions are available at little or no cost. Crack down on anti-competitive efforts to manipulate the patent system or collude on prices. Eliminate tax breaks for prescription drug advertisements."

<u>Complicating Factors</u>. The American health care cartel will prevent any financial harm from befalling one of its most prolific members. Drug prices are exorbitant by design. Nothing mints money quite like dealing drugs. Many, dare I say most health care stakeholders benefit from exorbitant drug prices alongside members of the pharmaceutical industry. It is easy to declare that Medicare will be empowered to negotiate. In reality, even if Medicare could negotiate as the VA does, there are no guarantees drug prices will come down since the American health care cartel will find a way to come out ahead. The American media industrial complex will also be at the forefront of those opposing the proposed elimination of tax breaks for prescription drug advertisements.

<u>Likely Outcomes</u>. I don't think the Democrats will find the votes to pass legislation empowering Medicare to negotiate for drugs. The pharmaceutical industry is a formidable and well-resourced opponent. If they see opposition approaching, they activate their army to neutralize the threat. Finally, even if a magic wand is waved and all the tactics are magically implemented, the American health care cartel will remain intact. And the American health care ecosystem will remain complex, expensive, and inequitable.

Proposed Solution 4: Reduce Health Care Costs and Improve Health Care Quality

<u>Tactics and Key Activities</u>
"Reduce out-of-pocket costs for families. Improve the quality

of health care for all. Ensure that no one pays more than 8.5-percent of their income in premiums. Eliminate the cap on subsidies. Outlaw surprise medical billing. Increase price transparency across all payers. Reduce paperwork through uniform medical billing. Use antitrust laws to fight against mega-mergers that would raise prices for patients by undermining market competition. Strengthen Medicare and fill coverage voids. Make it easier for every American to access preventive and primary health care."

Complicating Factors. Uncapped subsidies merely put more of the tab for the bloated American health care system on American taxpayers. Yet, many wonder why large corporations and wealthy individuals avoid paying federal tax like it's the plague. The American health care cartel will design loopholes into any attempts to abolish surprise medical billing. Antitrust laws are insufficient to stop market consolidation. In addition to undermining the antitrust enforcement workforce, the American health care cartel has several strategies to undermine market competition. For example, even if antitrust laws prevent a merger of two large hospital systems, one of the two hospital systems could decide to fail. There are many creative paths for hospital systems to take when they choose to die. Easiest is taking on unsustainable amounts of debt. Another is agreeing to be acquired by private equity funds who then load it up with unsustainable amounts of debt. In either scenario, the outcome is the same. Competition is eliminated. Strengthening Medicare and filling coverage voids will prove to be too costly. Clinician shortages and lengthy clinician development lifecycles will undermine efforts to expand preventive and primary health care access to all Americans.

Likely Outcomes. Though ambitious, I don't think most of what's proposed will actually be pursued in a meaningful way. I assume COVID-19 will remain the only health reform priority that gets any traction before the mid-term elections in 2022. The uncapping of subsidies is a handout to the American health care cartel, so I think that may actually go through. The payer community will be delighted. As we see with the Trump Administration's push for price transparency, the American health care cartel is successfully undermining that effort. I assume the Biden Administration won't fare any better. Finally, even if a magic wand is waved and all the tactics are magically implemented, the American health care cartel will remain intact. And the American health care ecosystem will remain complex, expensive, and inequitable.

Proposed Solution 5: Expand Access to Mental Health and Substance Use Treatment

Tactics and Key Activities

"Aggressively enforce the federal mental health parity law. Ensure that health insurers adequately cover mental health and substance use treatment. Invest in training and hiring more clinical and non-clinical mental health providers. Expand funding for health clinics, especially in rural areas. Increase access to mental health and substance use treatment services through Medicaid. Require publicly supported health clinics to offer Medication-Assisted Treatment (MAT) for opioid addiction. Make MAT available to all who need it. Expand access to mental health care in prisons and for returning citizens. Ensure no one is incarcerated solely for drug use."

Complicating Factors. Certain members of the American health care cartel will benefit from this. Others will not. The Congressional Budget Office (CBO) will likely deem the proposal as being too expensive. Creating capable and licensed mental health workers takes a very long time. This plan doesn't address the extended lifecycle. Many providers have stopped accepting Medicaid patients, so the impact of Medicaid expansion is limited. Though sometimes effective, promoting MAT is essentially a giveaway to the American health care cartel. Americans would be better off in the long run if those resources were directed towards addressing the root causes of opioid addiction instead of symptoms and consequences. The law enforcement industrial complex will also be at the forefront of those opposing the proposed elimination of incarceration for drug use.

Likely Outcomes. I don't think the authors of the proposed solution have sufficient appreciation for the extended lifecycle required to create capable and licensed mental health workers. Even with adequate insurance coverage, mental health worker capacity is limited. Medicaid coverage expansion as currently configured won't solve this problem. Finally, even if a magic wand is waved and all the tactics are magically implemented, the American health care cartel will remain intact. And the American health care ecosystem will remain complex, expensive, and inequitable.

Proposed Solution 6: Expand Long-Term Care Services and Supports

Tactics and Key Activities
"Eliminate state waiting lists for home and community-based care. Expand home care workforce. Develop a broader approach to eliminate the institutional bias within Medicaid. Improve nursing home staffing and quality standards. Strengthen accreditation processes. Combat corporate abuses in nursing homes. Prevent institutional segregation of people with disabilities."

Complicating Factors. The American health care cartel established state waiting lists for home and community-based care. They are also incentivized to keep the waiting lists long and convoluted. Many state governments will resist efforts to eliminate institutional bias within Medicaid. State governments mostly capitulate to the demands of the American health care cartel. It isn't a fair fight. Not even close. Reforming quality standards and accreditation processes will only benefit the quality measurement industrial complex. Incentives in the nursing home industry support an environment of corporate abuse and institutional segregation of people with disabilities.

Likely Outcomes. The American health care cartel will fight this every step of the way and likely prevent any meaningful change. State governments will probably never have sufficient tax revenue to meet the financial burden of expanding long-term care services and support. The federal government will pay the majority of this financial burden if this proposal is implemented. Finally, even if a magic wand is waved and all the tactics are magically implemented, the American health care cartel will remain intact. And the American health care ecosystem will remain complex, expensive, and inequitable.

Proposed Solution 7: Eliminate Racial, Gender, and Geographic Health Inequities

Tactics and Key Activities

"Launch a sustained, government-wide effort to eliminate racial, ethnic, gender, and geographic gaps in insurance rates, access to quality care, and health outcomes. Tackle the social, economic, and environmental inequities. Address social determinants of health like poor housing, hunger, inadequate transportation, mass incarceration, air and water pollution, and gun violence. Put environmental justice at the center of climate change and energy policies. Create a new environmental justice fund. Expand coverage. Make health care more affordable. Tackle implicit bias in the American health care system. Ensure federal data collection and analysis are adequately funded. Disaggregate federal data and analysis by race, gender, geography, disability status, etcetera. Invest significant new resources in clean water and wastewater infrastructure, clean energy generation, and distribution. Invest significant new resources in sustainable and regenerative agriculture. Significantly increase and make mandatory funding for the Indian Health Service. Restore federal funding for Planned Parenthood. Overturn federal and state laws that create barriers to women's reproductive rights. Repeal the Hyde Amendment. Protect and codify Roe v. Wade. Reauthorize the Violence Against Women Act. Reaffirm the rights of Indian tribes to prosecute anyone accused of

domestic violence and sexual assault on tribal lands. Increase resources to eliminate the national backlog of untested rape kits. Restore nondiscrimination protections for LGBTQ+ people in health insurance. Guarantee that LGBTQ+ people have full access to needed health care and resources. Require that federal health plans provide coverage for HIV/AIDS treatment and HIV prevention medications. Extend ACA coverage to Dreamers. Lift the five-year waiting period for Medicaid and Children's Health Insurance Program eligibility for low-income, lawfully present immigrants. Halt enforcement of the immigrant wealth test. Confront the epidemic of suicides-by-firearm. Ensure the Centers for Disease Control and Prevention have sufficient resources to study gun violence as a public health issue and support evidence-based programs for preventing gun violence."

<u>Complicating Factors</u>. There is no strategic approach to pursuing the expansive list of inequities this proposal wishes to resolve. Lists of tactics and key activities constructed in this manner are typically a catchall for items that aren't an absolute priority. Things that are considered a "long shot." The highest priorities will invariably be contaminated by demands included in the expansive list. Such contamination likely results in all the requests being denied outright or debated for years while Americans continue to suffer. I assume the divergent stakeholders who care about the different issues will fight to address their inequity first. There will be in-fighting and related conflict between marginalized communities. This proposal picks too many fights with too many different entrenched forces. The American health care cartel is more than enough to contend with. Attempting to pursue this proposal as currently configured won't end well. At least it won't end well for Americans and taxpayers.

<u>Likely Outcomes</u>. The American health care cartel will fight this every step of the way and prevent any meaningful reform of the inequities mentioned above. When groups take such a convoluted approach, I surmise they don't care about getting

any of their laundry list of loosely connected issues across the finish line. This proposal is too expensive. Way too expensive. Also, too many items are listed, so I won't attempt to parse my responses. In summary, even if a magic wand is waved and all the tactics are magically implemented, the American health care cartel will remain intact. And the American health care ecosystem will remain complex, expensive, and inequitable.

Proposed Solution 8: Strengthen and Support the Health Care Workforce

<u>Tactics and Key Activities</u>
"Ensure that all jobs in the caring economy come with family-sustaining wages, good benefits, access to training and professional development, and the ability to join a union and collectively bargain. Mandate all employers funded by taxpayer dollars pay their workers at least $15 an hour and protect workers' rights to organize. Invest in community health worker care-forces. Empower first-time mothers with nurse home visiting. Create a robust pipeline of talent with career ladders for work advancement. Increase opportunities for community health workers to come from the communities they serve."

<u>Complicating Factors</u>. There are many insurmountable challenges with this proposal. Employee wages and benefits have worsened over the years because the powers that be want it that way. The powers that be will not allow most workers to unionize and collectively bargain. Also, many unions have become corrupt cesspools. Implementing higher minimum wages will likely be viewed as too disruptive to the status quo. Finally, I'm not sure how the government will effectively mandate career advancement in private organizations.

<u>Likely Outcomes</u>. This proposal could have legs if the Biden Administration chooses to pursue it. However, the insurmountable challenges will remain insurmountable. The powers that be and the American health care cartel will undermine any effort to increase the minimum wage to $15 an

hour. They will also undermine efforts to enable worker unionization. Finally, even if a magic wand is waved and all the tactics are magically implemented, the American health care cartel will remain intact. And the American health care ecosystem will remain complex, expensive, and inequitable.

Proposed Solution 9: Invest in Health Science and Research

<u>Tactics and Key Activities</u>

"Support increased and sustainable funding for federal health and medical research across agencies. Increase federal investment in research and development for new medications and ensure a return on that investment for taxpayers. Increase funding for research into health disparities by race, gender, age, geographic area, and socioeconomic status. Focus on how the social determinants of health contribute to differences in health outcomes. Increase the diversity of principal investigators receiving federal grants. Increase the diversity of participants in federally-supported clinical trials. Improve the quality and applicability of medical research. Accelerate research into cancer and cancer treatments. Protect the independence and intellectual freedom of all scientists employed by the federal government or receiving federal grants supporting their research. Shield scientific research agencies from future political interference."

<u>Complicating Factors</u>. This reads like most of the others. Ambitious. Likely Dead on Arrival (DOA). Also, this proposal seeks to spend more money on the bloated American health care ecosystem without addressing the root causes driving its complexity, high prices, and inequities. **Side note:** Not quite sure I understand the utility of articulating proposals that have no chance of making it across the finish line. It's frustrating observing the investment of so much time and effort to achieve almost no progress. That's how the American health care cartel wants it, so I guess that's the way it is.

<u>Likely Outcomes</u>. Even if a magic wand is waved and all the tactics are magically implemented, the American health care

cartel will remain intact. And the American health care ecosystem will remain complex, expensive, and inequitable.

I'd like to give the Biden-Sanders unity task force health policy team the benefit of the doubt. However, I don't understand why they constructed their proposals in this manner. The document was clearly written to satisfy all the different constituents of the Democratic Party. How satisfying can it be to list tactics and activities on a piece of paper in a manner that makes it clear that the majority of the proposed efforts are DOA? Or equivalent to wishful thinking? There's no utility in being divorced from reality. None. It's just a distraction.

Health care policy recommendations from the 1% Steps for Health Care Reform project manifested similar issues. This effort also had a design flaw. It sought to identify small steps to reduce total health care spending. Akin to investing time and effort in acquiring buckets and hiring day laborers to displace water from an overflowing river. To avoid flooding in nearby towns and cities, I would suggest concentrating efforts on building dams and levees. Better yet, meaningfully address the human contributions to climate change, reducing the rate at which the earth's atmosphere is heating up, ultimately reducing rising water levels. Such efforts are more valuable than time and resources committed to lining the pockets of bucket manufacturers and enriching day laborers. Their labor should be invested in higher-value activities like the construction of dams and levees, not carrying buckets of water from an overflowing river. Anyway, I digress. I'll leave my environmental activism for another time.

Much of the 1% Steps for Health Care Reform project reads like a laundry list of wishes the American health care cartel would never grant. Wishes the political industrial complex and dominant market forces render infeasible. Other recommendations were essentially handouts to the American health care cartel. Handouts that weren't designed to make American health care simple, affordable, and equitable.

I have spoken with some of the health reform luminaries listed on the project website. I consider all of them respectable and informed. They are rational beings—esoteric knowledge experts for hire. Everyone has bills to pay. I get that. Yet, I struggle to understand why they think policymakers are scouring the internet looking for policy proposals. Whitepapers they can convert into a bill and enact into law.

Lobbyists and unelected staff members write the language that makes it into legislation.

Not lawmakers.

Surprising?

Not really.

It is by design.

According to the 1% Steps for Health Care Reform project website, the project is driven by the belief that there isn't a single thing wrong in the American health care ecosystem. Instead, differentially high health care spending in America results from a series of discrete problems that can and must be addressed. One by one. Baloney.

Swatting flies one by one without removing the horse manure attracting them is primarily a waste of time and energy. Attempts at reform should be focused on eliminating horse manure. Anything else is a distraction. These diversions are designed to pacify the masses by projecting that efforts to fundamentally improve the situation are on the horizon. They aren't. Incrementalism won't resolve this cancer. It can't.

Like playing a game of whack-a-mole, the American health care cartel ensures that every targeted effort to reduce spending in one area will result in comparable or higher expenditure elsewhere. This is the playbook. These luminaries know this. Yet, they pontificate about the impact of their proposed solutions on total health spending. I understand. Everyone has to eat. Wish they had more of an appetite for inherently higher-value meals.

The contributing authors to the 1% Steps for Health Care Reform project are overwhelmingly White and male. Typical. Only one Black person is featured on the website.

Tokenism? Mark, Zack, do better.

My dear friend Michael Chernew is a contributing author. Grateful he wrote the foreword to this book. Our relationship is as authentic as it gets. I shared my unfiltered feedback with him when the website first launched.

Yes.

I didn't pull any punches.

I'm not going to pull any punches.

Jason Abaluck and Johnathan Gruber believe structuring choice for health insurance plans will reduce total health spending by 0.63-percent. It won't. The political industrial complex and dominant market forces render the proposal infeasible. The American health care cartel won't allow it. Beyond that, there are other things I dislike about this proposal. It is merely an academic exercise. It doesn't even attempt to consider worsening market dynamics or the different ways the American health care cartel will respond. We don't live in a magical world where market forces are static. A world where affected stakeholders aren't using every tool in their toolkit to win.

Nikhil Agarwal, Itai Ashlagi, Michael Rees, and Alvin Roth believe expanding the kidney exchange will reduce total health spending by 0.02-percent. It won't. The political industrial complex and dominant market forces render the proposal infeasible. 0.02-percent. Really? I guess they were doing what they were hired to do. Propose seemingly low-hanging fruit. This proposal could help improve the supply of kidneys. However, the American health care cartel and interlopers involved in the kidney exchange will simply raise prices in the long run. Price increases that will eventually minimize or eliminate any projected savings.

Amitabh Chandra believes reforming the Orphan Drug Act (ODA) will reduce total health spending by 0.15-percent. It won't. The political industrial complex and dominant market forces render the proposal infeasible. The American health care cartel will never let that happen. Never. Not a chance. Elon Musk will build a Tesla on Mars with his bare hands before this proposal ever gets traction. No matter how tiny the projected savings. Any attempts to reform the ODA will only result in higher prices and expand therapies classified as orphan drugs. Unless we can dismantle the American health care cartel.

Michael Chernew, Leemore Dafny, and Maximilian Pany believe capping provider prices and price growth in the US commercial health sector will reduce total health spending by 1.8-percent. It won't. The political industrial complex and dominant market forces render the proposal infeasible. The American health care cartel won't allow it. I really wanted to like this one. For obvious reasons. Japan is an example of a national health care system that implemented a strategy of strict price controls. While they have mixed results over the years, Japanese people have one of the longest life expectancies in the world. Japan tightly regulates its health care ecosystem with stringent and sometimes punitive price controls. It's their ongoing strategy to rein in national health spending. The Japanese Ministry of Health negotiates rates with physicians every two years. Those negotiations determine the fee for every medical procedure and medication. Those fees are identical across the country. Japan has many different rules and idiosyncrasies designed into its health care ecosystem. Those peculiarities are absent from the American health care ecosystem. Merely cherry-picking and implementing one feature of their health care ecosystem gives me little reason to consider the estimated savings realizable. Why would providers ever agree to price caps? They hold all the cards in most health reform negotiations. They have sufficient market power to simply operate out-of-network. If antitrust enforcement is pursued, some providers will adopt the unsustainable debt strategy and eventually go out of business. Resulting in more consolidated markets. While payers will likely support this proposal, I assume that as more payers become payviders, that support will wane.

Zack Cooper and Fiona Scott Morton believe eliminating out-of-network billing policies will reduce total health spending by 1.67-percent. It won't. The political industrial complex and dominant market forces will make the projected savings unachievable. The American health care cartel will undermine it. The Whack-a-mole phenomenon is also at play here. Yet, on Dec. 27, 2020, the No Surprises Act was signed into law. While there are variances in the enacted law and the proposal from Zack and Fiona, we can put this in their win column. Most sections of the legislation go into effect on Jan. 1, 2022. Departments of Health and Human Services (HHS), Treasury, and Labor are tasked with issuing regulations and guidance to implement a number of the provisions. Departments of Transportation, Justice (DOJ), and the Federal Trade Commission (FTC) are also involved. I've witnessed first-hand how the process of implementing regulations and guidance can reimagine the intent of a law or provisions of law.

Further, there might be delays because HHS is required to coordinate with other agencies. Suppose the American health care cartel is sufficiently threatened by the rollout of this law. In that case, they will hire the regulators involved in drafting the implementing regulations to guide them by exploiting loopholes designed into the implementing rules. This law will undoubtedly introduce more complexity into the

American health care ecosystem. It will create additional opportunities for esoteric knowledge experts to extract more economic rents. The additional economic rents that flow to the esoteric knowledge experts will reduce the realizable savings. Finally, it is unlikely that HHS will have sufficient bandwidth or resources to audit all health plans for compliance with this law. Paying fines if and when caught for non-compliance is the American health care cartel's preferred strategy. Paid fines that ultimately get passed on to consumers. The penalties paid are almost always less than the economic rents extracted.

Zack Cooper and Martin Gaynor believe addressing hospital concentration and rising consolidation will reduce total health spending by 0.69-percent. It won't. The political industrial complex and dominant market forces render the proposal infeasible. The American health care cartel won't allow it. Market consolidation is a runaway train that can't be stopped. Antitrust laws remain ineffective. Increasing antitrust enforcement budgets could be helpful. However, increased budgets don't guarantee that DOJ and FTC will hire and retain capable human capital. The American health care cartel will likely never allow site-neutral billing to become law. If the government ever musters the political will to break up existing monopolies, the American health care cartel will wage an all-out war against such an effort. An all-out war they will win.

Leemore Dafny, Christopher Ody, and Matt Schmitt believe eliminating prescription drug copay coupons will reduce total health spending by 0.03-percent. It won't. The political industrial complex and dominant market forces render the proposal infeasible. The American health care cartel won't allow it. I guess 0.03-percent is better than 0.02-percent. Barely. Anyway, I digress. The pharmaceutical industry doesn't like to give up any ground. So I assume traction on this proposal will be hard. Likely impossible. While the target savings are minuscule, I don't think this policy proposal can realize the projected savings. It doesn't matter if the proposal is implemented as described. Whatever the pharmaceutical industry loses from a ban on prescription drug copay coupons will manifest as additional costs elsewhere. The American health care cartel has a well-rehearsed playbook to counteract these types of reform tactics.

Liran Einav, Amy Finkelstein, and Neale Mahoney believe eliminating the use of Long-Term Care Hospitals (LTCH) will reduce total health spending by 0.11-percent. It won't. The political industrial complex and dominant market forces render the proposal infeasible. The American health care cartel won't allow it. The administrative carve out that created LTCHs in the 1980s was designed to achieve the realized outcomes. Even if LTCHs were eliminated, something else would arise in its stead. The use of Skilled Nursing Facilities (SNFs) isn't ideal either. Long-term care should almost always be home-based. LTCHs are revered members of the American health care cartel—the worst of the worst. The scale of extraction of economic rent by LTCHs creates the type of balance sheet that can relentlessly "educate" countless legislators to look elsewhere for cost savings when health reform debates are underway.

Jonathan Gruber believes designing smart commercial insurer networks will reduce total health spending by 0.83-percent. It won't. The political industrial complex and dominant market forces render the proposal infeasible. The American health care cartel won't allow it. The nature of the policy recommendations in this proposal makes me wonder how Jonathan thinks market dynamics and stakeholder incentives will allow any of the projected savings to be realized. Offsets manifested in retaliatory price increases for "non-shoppable" services will only be the tip of the iceberg if this proposal is advanced. The myth of "shoppable" service will eventually fade once the monopolistic ambitions of the American health care cartel are fully implemented. I also dislike this proposal because it recommends shifting significant costs to patients—the powerless.

Daniel Kessler believes that increasing scrutiny of hospital ownership of physician practices will reduce total health spending by 0.91-percent. It won't. The political industrial complex and dominant market forces render the proposal infeasible. It doesn't matter if the FTC and DOJ increase antitrust scrutiny of vertically integrating physicians and hospitals. The American health care cartel will win that battle and every permutation that follows. I think these esoteric knowledge experts intuitively know this. But everyone has to eat, and this is the table they choose to dine on.

I could go on, but I am getting redundant.

I have been saying the same thing over and over again.

Apologies.

Covering my bases.

Stephen Lee and Jonathan Skinner believe that reforming home health care coverage to reduce fraud will reduce total health spending by 0.12-percent. It won't. The political industrial complex and dominant market forces render the proposal infeasible.

Mario Macis believes that removing all financial disincentives to living kidney donation will reduce total health spending by 0.08-percent. It won't. The political industrial complex and dominant market forces render the proposal infeasible.

Fiona Scott Morton believes that modifying the design of Medicare J-codes will generate competition amongst manufacturers of biologic Physician-Administered Drugs (PADs). She also believes that incentivizing physicians to prescribe lower-cost biosimilars in Medicare Part B will reduce total health spending by 0.21-percent. Implementing both ideas won't realize the projected savings. They can't. The political industrial complex and dominant market forces render the proposal infeasible.

Chima Ndumele—the only Black person on the website—and Jacob Wallace believe that improving auto-assignment in Medicaid Managed Care (MMC) will reduce total health spending by 0.24-percent. It won't. The political industrial complex and dominant market forces render the proposal infeasible.

Peter Orszag and Rahul Rekhi believe that real-time adjudication for health insurance claims will reduce total health spending by 1.25-percent. It won't. The political industrial complex and dominant market forces render the proposal infeasible. Wish I had more space to explain in excruciating detail why the American health care cartel will never let this fly. Unfortunately, this chapter is long enough as is.

Amanda Starc and Ashley Swanson believe that promoting preferred pharmacy networks will reduce total health spending by 0.04-percent. It won't. The political industrial complex and dominant market forces render the proposal infeasible.

All the ideas proposed on the website have some merit. However, absent any intervention, the cartel will always emerge victoriously. Always. Total health spending will increase. Complexity will increase. Patient suffering will increase. Given these realities, what's the point of all this work? The point to Americans and taxpayers that is. This work supports the livelihoods of esoteric knowledge experts. I guess that's the point. Hustle on, folks. I just wish you called out health reform horse manure more often, though.

I'd like to extend my gratitude to Yale University and Arnold Ventures for funding the work that went into the 1% Steps for Health Care Reform project website. It made it easier for me to find a broad spectrum of infeasible health reform proposals to critique. Infeasible since the political industrial complex and dominant market forces render all of the recommendations infeasible.

All of them.

Infeasible if the objective is reducing total health spending.

None of these will achieve that.

None of them.

Some of the listed proposals won't even reduce total health spending if successfully implemented, and the American health care cartel didn't exist. They do exist, though. That's the reality. I don't understand the utility of wishful thinking when trying to resolve cancer metastasizing at the intersection of White supremacy and American health care. Maybe that isn't the objective. That should be the objective.

While I appreciate the intellectual horsepower of the luminaries that developed the potential solutions I've examined in this chapter, they are merely esoteric knowledge experts in their selected niche areas.

They are satisficers and not maximizers.

They will never lead us to the "Promised Land."

Never.

Satisficers, by definition, pursue the minimum satisfactory condition or outcome. While that can be a prudent approach, it hasn't worked for health reform. It can't work for health reform. Esoteric knowledge experts have spent decades pontificating and satisficing.

Total health spending has exponentially grown in that time.

American health care has gotten more complex in that time.

Millions of Americans have continued to suffer in that time.

The minimum satisfactory outcome can't reduce total health spending.

It can't.

There appears to be a lack of authenticity shining through all the potential solutions. The authors are aware of the cartel's power. They know the cartel will block their solutions. Or undermine it. Yet, they propose and pontificate the infeasible.

If a solution is infeasible, why articulate it?

It is as helpful as being lost at sea with an expert diver and no scuba gear.

An expert pontificating about how having scuba gear could get you out of the crisis.

Pontificating when there is little chance scuba gear will ever materialize.

Pontificating while a shark fin is on the horizon.

Pontificating while you are drowning.

Pontificating while you are dying.

Pontificating after you're dead.

These luminaries are aware their proposals won't achieve the stated impact. Yet, they publish recommendations that won't accomplish the stated effects—reductions in total health spending. Maybe the stated effects are achievable in a magical kingdom. We live on earth, though. Narnia doesn't exist. Thankfully Turkish delights do. Anyway, I digress.

Esoteric knowledge experts are conditioned by the maneuvers of the cartel. As the adage goes, if someone is willing to pay…

They also want to continue extracting economic rents from the bloated American health care ecosystem instead of maximizing their potential by honing inherently valuable skills and pursuing alternative careers. I'm not knocking their hustle per se. Hard to teach an old dog new tricks. However, the harms of esoteric knowledge experts increasing the complexity of the

American health care ecosystem are real, pervasive, and long-lasting. Focus on adding value. Stop adding complexity.

Absent any paradigm-shifting interventions, total health spending will continue to increase. Exponentially. Given the current market dynamics and COVID-19, none of the policy proposals mentioned above can deter or delay that trend—none of them, including mine.

I remain perplexed by one lingering question.

Will enabling the creation of a more competitive and consumer-centric American health care ecosystem substantially reduce total health spending? I'm not sure. However, it is the best chance we have.

American prosperity continues to circle the drain when experts our leaders turn to don't speak truth to power while the American health care cartel continues to laugh all the way to the bank.

The American health care ecosystem <u>isn't broken</u>.

It isn't damaged. It can't be fixed.

It is <u>designed</u> like other American institutions.

Designed to prioritize the needs of wealthy White males.

Designed to deprioritize the needs of people who aren't White.

<u>Designed to uphold the legacy of White supremacy in America</u>.

That's the <u>truth</u>.

The whole <u>truth</u>.

Nothing but the <u>truth</u>.

"Nothing is impossible." – Aliko Dangote

Actualizing Paradigm-shifting Change

"Change will not come if we wait for some other person or some other time. We are the ones we've been waiting for. We are the change we seek." – President Barack Obama

Throughout history, a crisis has forced humans to break with the past and reimagine their world. <u>Arresting and resolving cancer metastasizing at the intersection of White supremacy and American health care requires a similar approach</u>.

<u>We the People</u> of these United States must enable a redesign of the American health care ecosystem. The reimagined ecosystem will deliver more value for patients and taxpayers. To achieve this feat, Americans must reject fascists preoccupied with calcifying the cancer of White supremacy in America. Fascists whose words and deeds accelerate the decay of American prosperity.

Decay of America's relevance around the world.

<u>Americans must choose a more prosperous path</u>. Establishing American institutions designed to enable American prosperity is the more prosperous path. We must establish institutions that work for all Americans. Not just wealthy White males, oligarchs, and their cronies.

When I embrace my cynical mindset, I assume America is actually under one-party rule. A single party with two flavors. The two Parties are rendering similar services while donning different masks. Both were designed to empower and enrich White males, American oligarchs, and their cronies. My cynical mindset assumes the two Parties serve the same master.

Protecting corporate profits.

Upholding White supremacy.

That's their master.

Spinning stories designed to mesmerize exhausted masses into believing either of the two Parties is committed to improving their life outcomes.

Topher Spiro challenged that cynical mindset. We met in the fall of 2016. At the time we met, Topher was the Vice President responsible for the health care portfolio at the Liberal think tank, Center for American Progress (CAP). We met in a conference room at CAP headquarters. One of his female colleagues accompanied him. I don't remember her name.

In 2021, the Biden Administration appointed Topher as the Principal Associate Director (PAD) for the health programs portfolio at the White House Office of Management and Budget (OMB). The health program PAD is responsible for the trillion-dollar portfolio that oversees federal spending in programs like Medicare and Medicaid.

We met to discuss strategies capable of meaningfully bending the cost curve of American health care without undermining health care quality or outcomes. I was still in my role at the Laura and John Arnold Foundation at the time. Meetings are always easier to schedule when you are in an influential position. Anyway, I digress.

During the meeting, I shared a concept I thought could become viable at scale. The idea I shared was the same one I shared with Farzad Mostashari earlier that fall. The idea was a combination of Professor Michael Porter's Centers-of-Excellence (CoE) strategy and medical tourism.

Topher questioned the viability of the strategy by opining that Medicare fee schedules are the same across America. He wondered what incentive people would have to travel to CoE sites to receive care. I explained how regional and local market dynamics determined the actual reimbursement rates providers can demand and often receive in health care markets across America.

Two things struck me in our conversation. First, I wondered how one of the smartest guys in the room, when the Affordable Care Act (ACA) was crafted, wasn't fully aware of regional and geographic variations in Medicare fee schedules or reimbursement rates.

While I acknowledge that no single individual can know everything about American health care, I assumed a meaningful understanding of regional and geographic variations were table-stakes. Essential knowledge for folks committed to meaningfully reforming the American health care ecosystem.

I was mistaken.

Second, as I explained to Topher how members of the American health care cartel hired esoteric knowledge experts to design strategies to undermine the ACA and exploit loopholes in the enacted law, he seemed genuinely surprised to hear what I was explaining to him.

I was surprised by his surprise.

I assumed everyone around the table when the ACA was being crafted was in on the hustle. I was mistaken. Based on Topher's reaction, it would appear that some folks around the table weren't aware of what was fundamentally transpiring.

The American health care cartel strikes again.

American prosperity decays.

While I briefed him about some consulting work I did for the American health care cartel, his demeanor gave me hope. The hope challenged my cynical mindset that assumed influential people on both sides of the aisle served the same master. As we wrapped the meeting, he suggested we talk to Farzad and Zeke Emanuel about the concept I shared with him. I let him know that when I spoke with Farzad, he wasn't keen on shifting his attention from his current ACO-centric plans to scale Aledade.

Topher suggested we stay in touch and find time to chat with Farzad and Zeke. That group conversation never happened. Hillary Clinton lost the 2016 presidential election a few weeks after our meeting. I haven't spoken to Topher since.

There are several reasons why both Parties that dominate Congress receive low approval ratings routinely. Many Americans view Congress as a group of politicians who are out of touch with their constituents. Instead of enacting the people's will, some of the politicians in Congress are preoccupied with political theater, bestowing favor on special interest groups and designing schemes to protect corporate profits.

Congress is the pinnacle of institutionalized White mediocrity. Congress continues to elevate White mediocrity above establishing a more equitable American democracy. From Rep. Matt Gaetz to Rep. Marjorie Taylor Greene, White "dudes" and "dudettes" run wild. Embarrassing the nation with their words and deeds. Like caged primates flinging feces, White "dudes" and "dudettes" in Congress are easy to observe in their artificial habitat. They are often found flinging rhetoric and committing atrocities unbecoming of the offices they hold. Wielding power to make laws and allocate taxpayer resources. Manifesting White privilege in its most insidious form.

Both Parties have their fair share of mediocre underperformers and sordid histories. Their sordid pasts are full of policies and laws that strengthened White supremacy's stranglehold on American society. The current Republican Party has chosen a strategy that propagates White supremacy and embraces fascism. They have chosen an approach to lay the foundation for a nation dominated politically, socially, and economically by the nation's eventual minority White population.

They want to establish apartheid in America. That's their plan. They have chosen a strategy that empowers mediocre White "dudes" to continue dragging this great nation towards irrelevance.

The Republican Party gave America President Abraham Lincoln, who abolished slavery and enacted the emancipation proclamation. Unfortunately, the Republican Party also gave America White "dudes" like President Ronald Reagan and President Donald Trump. President Reagan started the "War on Drugs," which should have the more appropriate title, "manufacturing fodder for the law enforcement industrial complex." President Reagan's "War on Drugs" has done more to destabilize more American families and traumatize young American children than all the rap videos ever created could. In 10 lifetimes. President Trump mishandled the federal response to COVID-19. A calamity that resulted in almost half a million American lives lost to COVID-19 during his tenure. Also, given its disdain for Hollywood celebrity culture and mainstream media, I find it a tad ironic that the Republican Party is the political institution that elevated a washed-up actor and a reality TV villain to the most powerful position in America.

The current Democratic Party seems to be pursuing an inclusive, pro-democracy agenda. However, it's hard to forget that the Democratic Party gave America the infamous pro-segregation, racist Governor, George Wallace. The Democratic Party also controlled southern states that sought to secede from the union—the precursor to the civil war. Southern states sought to secede in a bid to uphold and expand the barbaric practice of human chattel slavery.

Fortunately, the Democratic Party also gave America President Lyndon B. Johnson. He enacted multiple civil rights laws and established the Medicare and Medicaid programs. The Democratic Party also gave America President Barack H. Obama. He enacted the Affordable Care Act.

Most recently, the Democratic Party has given the nation President Joseph R. Biden. A president who seems to be pursuing an ambitious policy agenda designed to address the concerns of all Americans. He doesn't appear to be preoccupied with the concerns of wealthy White males, oligarchs, and their cronies.

While both parties are articulating divergent paths for the future of America, the American health care cartel continues to wield its power over the political industrial complex.

The American health care cartel is poised to maintain its power.

Power over the political industrial complex.

Regardless of which political Party is in power.

The American health care ecosystem remains on a path that promotes complexity, excessive spending, and worsening health disparities.

A path destined to undermine American prosperity.

Campaign finance corruption, partisan gerrymandering, and voter suppression laws strengthen the American health care cartel's grip on the political industrial complex.

Fortunately, all hope is not lost because <u>pro-democracy Americans</u> still have the voters and the real power in our crumbling democracy.

The power necessary to abolish the political industrial complex.

Successfully abolishing the political industrial complex is the <u>only way</u> to loosen the American health care cartel's stranglehold on American prosperity. It is the only way to arrest and resolve harmful, uncompetitive market dynamics.

Reimagining America's political infrastructure <u>will resolve</u> cancer metastasizing at the intersection of White supremacy and American health care. Cancer enabled by campaign finance corruption, partisan gerrymandering, and voter suppression laws.

An effectively redesigned American political infrastructure must ensure that all Americans have equitable access to cast their vote. It must enable the election of competent leaders who are capable of <u>enacting the will of the people</u>.

Effectively redesigning America's political infrastructure requires pro-democracy Americans to embrace a strategic migration playbook to strengthen America's democracy.

A strategic migration agenda to save America.

A strategic migration agenda to maximize the potential of all Americans.

A strategic migration agenda to liberate America from the tyranny of White supremacy.

A strategic migration agenda to establish America as a pro-democracy nation.

To win, pro-democracy Americans must organize, mobilize, and migrate to states where their votes will have the most significant impact. America's political infrastructure was designed to propagate the dominance of its White male minority over the masses.

That infrastructure is strengthened after every election cycle.

In its formative years, the combination of America's population of indigenous people and enslaved people from Africa was more significant than its population of White males. With surgical precision, America's White "dudes" slaughtered and exiled indigenous Americans. Those indigenous Americans were exiled to Central and South America. America's White "dudes" dehumanized, mutilated, and murdered American-born descendants of people forcibly removed from Africa.

To swell their ranks, America's White "dudes" imported additional White people from Europe. While many European imports still struggled to find their place in American society, many were given access to resources withheld from recently emancipated Americans. Emancipated Americans that were descendants of enslaved people from Africa.

Pro-democracy Americans, specifically those represented in Table 1, must <u>flee</u> from states where pro-democracy votes won't matter for the foreseeable future.

Table 1: States where pro-democracy American votes are being wasted

2020 Election	Pro-democracy Votes	Loss Margin Percentage	Electoral College	2021 Maternal Mortality Rate	COVID-19 Death Rate
Puerto Rico*	1,500,000	N/A	0	N/A	758 (45th)
West Virginia	235,984	-38.9%	5	12.9 (13th)	1,535 (31st)
Arkansas	423,932	-27.6%	6	37.5 (46th)	1,916 (18th)
Kentucky	772,474	-25.9%	8	22.9 (36th)	1,486 (34th)
Alabama	849,624	-25.5%	9	36.4 (45th)	2,244 (10th)
Louisiana	856,034	-18.6%	8	58.1 (50th)	2,252 (8th)
Mississippi	539,508	-16.5%	6	20.8 (30th)	2,435 (5th)
Indiana	1,242,413	-16.1%	11	43.6 (48th)	1,998 (13th)
Missouri	1,253,014	-15.4%	10	34.6 (44th)	1,510 (32nd)
TOTAL	7,672,983		63		N/A

*Puerto Rico is a U.S. territory where millions of Americans live. They have no Senators or Electoral College votes. I assume 1.5 million of the more than 3 million residents of Puerto Rico will likely vote for a Democratic ticket.
Note: Election results data - https://cookpolitical.com/2020-national-popular-vote-tracker
Rate/100,000 births - Maternal Mortality Rate By State 2021 (worldpopulationreview.com) 5/14/21
Death/1 million - https://www.kff.org/other/state-indicator/cumulative-covid-19-cases-and-deaths (5/14/21)

States that have doubled down on upholding White supremacy. States with higher rates of moms dying during childbirth. States where Black moms suffer the most. States well represented in the 10 worst states for maternal mortality. States well represented in the 10 worst states for COVID-19 deaths. Alabama and Louisiana must be avoided. Both states have the dishonor of being featured in both 10-worst lists of states for maternal mortality and COVID-19 deaths.

Pro-democracy Americans, specifically those represented in Table 1, must migrate to battleground states listed in Table 2. Battleground states President Biden won by relatively slim margins in 2020. To strengthen our democracy, pro-democracy Americans must reinforce those states and help retain the Electoral College coalition that put President Biden in the White House.

Table 2: States where pro-democracy American votes need immediate reinforcements

2020 Election	Pro-democracy Win Margin	Win Margin %	Electoral College	Senate Seats
Pennsylvania	80,555	1.2%	20	2
Georgia	11,779	0.2%	16	2
Michigan	154,188	2.8%	16	2
Arizona	10,457	0.3%	11	2
Wisconsin	20,682	0.6%	10	2
Nevada	33,596	2.4%	6	2
TOTAL	311,257		79	12

Note: Election results data - https://cookpolitical.com/2020-national-popular-vote-tracker

Pro-democracy Americans, specifically those represented in Table 3, must maintain a voting-eligible presence in multiple states. If they can afford to do so. They must establish a secondary residence in battleground states listed in Table 2. Pro-democracy Americans that reside in the states listed in Table 3 must embrace the tradition of elite migrating snowbirds. Elite migrating snowbirds enjoy the privilege of casting their ballots in states where their votes can significantly impact presidential elections and national bellwether policies. These pro-democracy Americans must also establish new battleground states from the list of states in Table 4.

Table 3: States with an overabundance of pro-democracy American votes being wasted

2020 Election	Pro-democracy Win Margin	Win Margin %	Electoral College	Senate Seats
California	5,103,821	29.2%	55	2
New York	1,992,889	23.1%	29	2
Massachusetts	1,215,000	33.5%	11	2
Illinois	1,025,024	17.0%	20	2
Maryland	1,008,609	33.2%	10	2
Washington D.C.*	298,737	86.8%	3	0
TOTAL	**10,644,080**		**128**	**10**

*Washington D.C. isn't recognized as a State. It should be. White supremacy at work. Infuriating

Note: Election results data - https://cookpolitical.com/2020-national-popular-vote-tracker

Pro-democracy Americans, particularly those represented in Tables 1 and 3, must migrate to or establish secondary residences in states President Biden lost by a narrow vote count margin.

Pro-democracy Americans must strategically establish a voting-eligible presence in states with the highest Electoral College Per Capita™ impact.

States that can be converted and reestablished.

States that can be pro-democracy.

American citizens, families, communities, organizations, and governmental entities all play an essential role in implementing a strategic migration playbook to strengthen America's democracy. Pro-democracy citizens and entities should explore various tactics to identify which approach best fits them and their situation.

<u>Pro-democracy American citizens, families, and communities</u> who currently reside in locations listed in Table 1 should flee to their preferred states listed in Table 2. They can work remotely if they aren't able to find a job in their new home state.

Table 4: States that can be reimagined with a modest infusion of pro-democracy American voters

2020 Election	Pro-democracy Loss Margin	Loss Margin %	Electoral College	Per Capita	Senate Seats
North Carolina	74,483	-1.3%	15	4,966	2
Alaska	36,173	-10.1%	3	12,058	2
Florida	371,686	-3.4%	29	12,816	2
Iowa	138,611	-8.2%	6	23,102	2
South Carolina	293,562	-11.7%	9	32,618	2
Montana	98,816	-16.4%	3	32,939	2
Kansas	201,083	-14.7%	6	33,514	2
South Dakota	119,572	-26.2%	3	39,857	2
North Dakota	120,693	-33.4%	3	40,231	2
Wyoming	120,068	-43.4%	3	40,023	2
Idaho	267,098	-40.0 %	4	66,775	2
TOTAL	**1,832, 845**		**84**		**22**

*Electoral College Per Capita™ is derived by dividing Biden Loss Margin votes by the number of Electoral College votes in each State. Electoral College Per Capita™ impact is determined by how few additional pro-democracy Americans per Electoral College vote are required to establish a pro-democracy majority in any State.
** Crude math. I'm aware. Hopefully, it got my point across.
Note: Election results data - https://cookpolitical.com/2020-national-popular-vote-tracker

<u>Retired pro-democracy Americans</u> currently residing in states listed in Tables 1 or 3 should relocate or establish a secondary residence in their preferred states listed in Table 2.

<u>Pro-democracy corporations, non-governmental organizations, and government entities</u> should institute permanent remote work policies. They should establish employee co-working hubs in the states listed in Table 2. Once states listed in Table 2 secure adequate pro-democracy win margins, they can replicate the same strategy in states listed in Table 4.

<u>Pro-democracy Medicare Advantage (MA) plans</u> that aren't card-carrying members of the American health care cartel should establish affordable senior living hubs for their members residing in states listed in Table 2. Those senior living

hubs should have wraparound services that address Social Drivers of Health (SDoH). MA plans should encourage their members residing in locations listed in Table 1 to migrate to states listed in Table 2. They should concentrate their efforts in one state listed in Table 2.

I would recommend Georgia.

Hang in there Stacey, reinforcements are on the way.

<u>Pro-democracy entrepreneurs</u> currently residing in locations listed in Table 3 should migrate to states listed in Table 4. They should start new businesses in the states listed in Table 4. The new companies should reinvent the state and attract more pro-democracy Americans.

Pro-democracy Americans that choose to embark on this mission will be joining a growing coalition of American maximizers and justice activists.

The time to act is now!

Pro-democracy Americans have a <u>shrinking window of opportunity</u> to successfully complete this mission. Fascists appointed and elevated by the Trump Administration made their intentions known in the Administration's waning months.

War-gaming exercises are valuable when establishing strategic playbooks. This situation is no different. I've stress-tested the strategic migration playbook.

It is almost impossible to defeat.

Fascists can't defeat it.

The only thing that defeats the strategic migration playbook is if pro-democracy Americans don't organize, mobilize, migrate, and vote.

We can do it.

Let's get it done!

Fascists preoccupied with laying a foundation for apartheid in America won't have an effective countermove. If they abolish the Electoral College, pro-democracy Americans will win the popular vote by a landslide. Forever.

If they abolish snow-birding, that will hurt wealthy anti-democracy Americans more.

Even if they abolish the Electoral College, successful implementation of the strategic migration playbook will empower pro-democracy Americans to capture greater representation in both chambers of Congress. Capture greater representation across state legislatures.

Pro-democracy Americans must amend the Constitution of the United States.

We must secure two-thirds of the seats in Congress.

We must secure three-fourths of state legislatures.

We can do it.

We must do it.

The future we seek depends on it.

Amending the United States Constitution is how we defeat fascism, White supremacy, and the American health care cartel. It is the only way.

The one and only.

If fascist rulers ever get another chance to control both chambers of Congress and the Office of the President, American democracy and its institutions will be destroyed.

Yes.

Destroyed.

Fascists aren't yucking around.

They mean business.

Always.

Yuck!

Fascist rulers have many insidious objectives. Their most detrimental plan for American democracy is the politicization and dumbing-down of the leadership ranks of the federal civil service.

The Trump Administration attempted to implement rules that would have made it easier to fire and replace influential senior civil servants like Dr. Anthony Fauci. Influential senior civil servants that President Trump wanted to permanently replace with mediocre White "dudes" like the pillow guy.

A federal government unified under fascist rule across both chambers of Congress and the President's Office will usher in a wave of widespread installation of political hacks and grafters into the most influential senior civil service positions. A tide of White mediocrity that will exacerbate America's vulnerabilities at home and abroad.

Lest we forget, millions of Americans have suffered and continue to suffer from preventable calamities initiated during the Bush and Trump Administrations.

Americans suffered through the deadly terrorist attacks that occurred on 9/11. Americans suffered through the abysmal federal response to Hurricane Katrina in Louisiana. Americans suffered through a subprime mortgage loan crisis that plunged millions of American families into financial ruin. Preventable calamities and needless American suffering actualized during the 8-years President George W. Bush was in power.

Such preventable calamities and needless suffering caused many to commit suicide.

Similarly, during the Trump Administration, Americans suffered through the abysmal federal response to Hurricane

Maria in Puerto Rico. Americans are still suffering from the deadly COVID-19 pandemic. A pandemic that could have been managed competently by the Trump Administration if they had more competent people placed in positions of authority. A mismanaged pandemic that caused many Americans to suffer through an economic recession.

Both Administrations had something in common.

An overabundance of mediocre White "dudes" and "dudettes" appointed to positions of authority across the federal government.

The perils of elevating mediocrity are real and long-lasting.

We still have Americans needlessly dying on foreign soil.

Trapped in meaningless conflicts that the Bush Administration started over a decade ago.

Preventable calamities cause Americans to suffer needlessly.

Acting now provides pro-democracy Americans a fighting chance to effectively abolish the political industrial complex. Once vanquished, we can loosen the stranglehold the American health care cartel has on American prosperity.

If we don't, American prosperity will continue to rot.

Increasing rates of Indebtedness.

Hopelessness.

Stress.

Chronic illness.

Mental illness.

Declining life expectancy and birth rates.

Yeah.

Rot is apt.

Abolishing the political industrial complex and reimagining America's political infrastructure will require more contributions from American maximizers and justice activists.

Organizing, mobilizing, migrating, and voting are table-stakes.

American maximizers and justice activists must be elected.

They must pursue civil service careers.

Pro-democracy super-majorities must be achieved in both chambers of Congress.

Super-majorities must be achieved across state legislatures.

We can do this.

We can save America.

American maximizers and justice activists must be elected.

They must be appointed to positions of authority.

Then, <u>We the People</u> will be empowered to abolish the political industrial complex.

Like a phoenix rising from its ashes, the reimagined political infrastructure that rises from the ashes of the political industrial complex must be reimagined to equitably serve all Americans.

The reimagined political infrastructure must abolish campaign finance corruption, partisan gerrymandering, and voter suppression laws.

Reimagined campaign finance rules must <u>ban organizations from financing election campaigns</u>. Corporations aren't individuals. Only individuals are individuals. Only individuals should have First Amendment rights. Only individuals must be legally allowed to contribute to election campaigns.

The Citizen's United decision must be overturned.

Lower individual contribution limits must be established and enforced.

A reimagined political infrastructure must <u>abolish partisan gerrymandering</u>. All district boundary lines must be redrawn by nonpartisan, independent commissions. Nonpartisan, independent commissions staffed by unelected Americans that reside in different communities across each state.

Elected officials must be prohibited from participating in redistricting.

They must.

It is the only way.

All district boundary lines must be redrawn to create geographically proximal enclaves that loosely resemble recognizable shapes like rectangles and squares—shapes with no tributaries or protrusions designed to convey partisan advantage.

A reimagined political infrastructure must <u>abolish voter suppression laws</u>.

Election days must be established as federal holidays. Americans must have convenient avenues to cast their votes.

We can make this a reality. Our reality.

Only if we organize, mobilize, migrate, and vote like our lives depended on it.

Our lives depend on it.

Our livelihoods depend on it.

Our children's lives depend on it.

The reimagined political infrastructure <u>may</u> have the following features:

This list of potential features of a reimagined political infrastructure is an opening salvo. Absent any intervention, fascists and the American health care cartel can cancel some of these features.

We the People can invent a future where they can't.

We the People, will ultimately decide the final list of features.

Features we want in a reimagined American political infrastructure.

1. <u>Publicly-funded mass media platform</u>. All election campaign advertisements will be aired and distributed on a dedicated, publicly-funded mass media platform. No exceptions. Privately-funded campaign advertisements promoting or smearing specific candidates or policies will be abolished. Candidates who violate this rule will be disqualified. Privately-funded advertisements providing nonpartisan information about where and how to vote will be permitted. All election-related advertisements will be fact-checked by Election authorities before dissemination. All candidates authorized to participate in an election cycle will receive equal airtime on the publicly-funded mass media platform.

2. <u>Mandatory capability assessments</u>. All candidates pursuing public office will be required to publicly complete written capability assessments across three domains. The three domains will be civics, empathy, and decision-making. Assessment results will be publicly revealed upon completion. Candidate results and responses will be discussed instead of traditional debate questions. NFL teams that primarily exist to entertain Americans require their potential employees to undergo rigorous evaluation, including the Wonderlic assessment.

Yet, Americans elect candidates without any insight into critical pieces of information.

We elect those candidates into positions of authority over our lives.

We elect them to be the stewards of American democracy.

Upholders of western democracy.

<u>We the People</u>, don't care how many corn-dogs a candidate can stuff in their face at the Iowa fair.

<u>We the People</u>, don't care how many rehearsed lines they can spew during a debate.

<u>We the People</u>, deserve to know how civic-minded they are.

How empathetic to the needs of all Americans they are.

What framework they use to make decisions.

All public servants and civil servants must be required to complete similar assessments.

3. <u>Modern election infrastructure</u>. We will establish an accelerated timeline to eventually sunset paper ballots and mail-in-voting. We will embrace emerging technologies like Distributed Ledger Technology (DLT) to modernize the entire voting ecosystem.

    Results will be authenticated efficiently. Effectively.

    User data will be secure and encrypted.

    Polling data and projections will be more precise. Post-election analysis and insights will be instantaneous and more accurate.

4. <u>6-year presidential term</u>. Presidents will only get one term. Hopefully, they make it count. The current 4-year, two-term design is inefficient. Ineffective. Prioritizes re-

election campaign posturing and deprioritizes good governance.

It traumatizes civil servants.

Most Administrations are typically only fully functional for 2-years out of each 4-year term. The first year is preoccupied with onboarding political appointees. The fourth year is consumed with re-election campaigning, political appointee job-hunting, or burrowing.

One 6-year presidential term is a better value for presidents and taxpayers.

Better for Americans. That's the pro-democracy way.

5. <u>4-year terms in the House of Representatives</u>. 2-years is insufficient. Especially with current prolonged election lifecycles and fundraising requirements. 4-year terms will likely encourage voters and political institutions to rigorously evaluate candidates they choose to elect to the House of Representatives. Hopefully.

6. <u>25-year term limits for public servants</u>. No one will serve in Congress for more than 25 consecutive years. No one.

Lifetime appointments will be abolished.

The 25-year term limit will be extended to the U.S. Supreme Court and the rest of the federal judiciary. 25-year term limits will discourage the appointment of inappropriate candidates to the U.S. Supreme Court and across the federal judiciary. Every public servant will be encouraged to retire at some point in their careers.

There's no nobility in dying on that job.

None.

Why should the rest of us suffer because some people wish to die on the job? I understand why families may not want these people to spend more time at home. Or maybe they're estranged. Not our problem.

In any event, they should leave us alone and get a hobby.

Or a pet.

Or something.

Just leave us alone.

7. <u>Reformed federal judiciary</u>. The number of U.S. Supreme Court justices will align with the number of circuit court systems in the federal judiciary.

    Yes, I'm aware there are 13 circuit court systems.

    All federal justices will be required to complete annual competency assessments after the age of 75. Failure to comply or failure to achieve a satisfactory assessment score will result in automatic impeachment and removal from the federal judiciary.

    Removal decisions will be final and not subject to appeal.

    Come on. Justices, you're over 75.

    You've had a good run.

    Enjoy retirement.

    Or not.

    Just leave us alone.

8. <u>Simplified path to statehood</u>. American districts and territories with more than 300,000 American residents will be granted statehood. States with less than 300,000 American residents will lose statehood.

    More than 300,000 Americans cast their ballots in the District of Columbia.

The District of Columbia will become a state.

They will get two Senate seats.

They will get equitable representation in the House of Representatives.

More than 3 million Americans live in Puerto Rico. They aren't allowed to vote in presidential elections. They aren't represented in Congress. Puerto Rico will become a state. Puerto Rico will get two Senate seats and equitable representation in the House.

States with more than 20 million residents will be required to split into two states.

Yes, split.

Like the Dakotas.

Or the Carolinas.

Split states will proportionally allocate Electoral College votes.

Each split state will maintain two Senate seats.

According to the U.S. Census Bureau, more than 39 million people live in California. More than 29 million people live in Texas. More than 21 million people live in Florida. More than 20 million people live in New York. All four states will be split. Newly established states will include:

North California and South California.

North Texas and South Texas.

North Florida and South Florida.

North New York and South New York.

They can also opt to split East to West.

Pro-democracy state legislatures will decide.

9. <u>Shortened election lifecycles</u>. A single 3-month period will be dedicated to all election-related activities. Elected officials will spend the majority of their time governing and engaging their constituents. Elected officials will stop spending a majority of their time groveling at the feet of donors, lobbyists, and political "kingmakers."

10. <u>Permanent ban on lobbying</u>. Lobbying will be reclassified as what it actually is, bribery.

    Bribery will become a capital crime.

    Yes, bribery, formerly known as lobbying, will become a capital crime.

    The catastrophic impact of bribery is multi-generational.

    It fundamentally betrays the democratic process.

    Undermines the will of the people.

    Millions of American lives and livelihoods have been destroyed by the negative externalities of bribery. Adequate federal appropriations will be made available for Congress to acquire unbiased, evidence-based information on any topic or issue policymakers want to be educated on. The Executive Branch will be authorized to draft legislative language for Congress to review, markup, and propose in either chamber of Congress.

11. <u>Open primaries and ranked-choice voting</u>. Partisan extremism will be reduced or eliminated. Candidates will be incentivized to appeal to a broad array of the electorate, not just the fringe. Voter participation will increase.

Pro-democracy Americans must unite and elect at least one pro-democracy senator capable of ruthlessly executing a long-term pro-democracy agenda. Congress needs pro-democracy senators capable of functioning as a counterbalance to Senator Mitch McConnell.

Or politicians being groomed to replace him after he dies in office.

My money is on Senator Josh Hawley.

Senator Mitch McConnell is a masterclass in long-term political strategy execution.

In the past 20-years, he has been ruthlessly implementing the fascist plan of establishing a foundation for apartheid in America. Pro-democracy Americans need to elect at least one senator capable of ruthlessly establishing and executing a long-term, pro-democracy plan for America. That long-term, pro-democracy agenda must include pathways to resolving America's worsening partisan divide.

Divided, we decay.

American prosperity rots.

United, we stand.

Better together.

Stronger together.

Americans must learn to peaceably co-exist with people they disagree with.

We must learn to peaceably co-exist with people we cannot relate to.

We must focus on maximizing the potential of every American.

Maximized potential enhances America's paths to prosperity.

America's real enemies aren't Americans.

Our real enemies are fascists who want to undermine America's role in the world.

Our role as a stronghold for democratic ideals.

America's real enemies are Communist Chinese imperialists and Russian oligarchs. Authoritarian regimes frightened by the potential of an America liberated from the tyranny of White mediocrity in positions of authority. A nation poised to maximize its true potential.

An America finally poised to <u>become that fabled shining city on a hill</u>.

A shining city on a hill capable of <u>giving oppressed masses around the world hope</u>.

Hope that the will of the people can matter.

Hope that the masses can overcome their oppressors.

Hope for a better life and future for their children.

Hope for a fair and benevolent government.

Hope that the color of a person's skin, gender, sexual orientation, or religious preference doesn't condemn them to an existence defined by discrimination and marginalization.

A reimagined political infrastructure establishes an equitable, merit-based democracy that will elect capable leaders to enact the people's will. Paradigm-shifting ideas can be ignited with a reimagined political infrastructure.

Paradigm-shifting ideas can be successfully implemented.

They can evolve American health care into a simple, affordable, and equitable ecosystem.

They can dismantle the American health care cartel.

They can bolster American prosperity.

Implementing paradigm-shifting ideas will help establish a simple, affordable, and equitable American health care ecosystem.

A health care ecosystem that doesn't undermine American prosperity.

Some paradigm-shifting ideas were explored in the previous chapter on potential solutions. Pushing the envelope farther, I'm highlighting a shortlist of additional paradigm-shifting ideas I'd recommend we prioritize.

Paradigm-shifting ideas that can meaningfully improve American health care.

1. Establish and enforce stringent anti-cartel regulations. Abolishing and prosecuting all anti-competitive agreements will weaken the American health care cartel. Abolishing and prosecuting all abuses by dominant health care stakeholders creates disincentives. Proverbial sticks that will curtail escalating violations by the American health care cartel. Eliminating caps on the punitive damages awarded to parties harmed by cartels will financially terrify the American health care cartel. Establishing mandatory minimums and lengthy prison sentences for individuals guilty of violating anti-cartel regulations will psychologically terrify the American health care cartel. Hopefully, the publicized take-downs of bad actors and threats of enforcement action will scare the American health care cartel straight.

2. Eliminate fee-for-service transaction architecture. Fee-for-service contracting and transactions are the foundation and fuel for the unnecessary complexity that plagues the American health care ecosystem. Enacting laws banning the use of fee-for-service transaction architecture and contracting will incentivize new entrants and incumbents to build and scale viable alternatives. Distributed Ledger Technology (DLT) is a promising Alternative Payment Model (APM) architecture. Adopting DLT as an APM platform will

streamline, automate, and simplify transaction execution. That transformation also dramatically reduces transaction costs. In addition to significantly reduced technology costs, it will no longer be necessary to employ hordes of esoteric knowledge experts and interlopers. Complex fee-for-service transactions will no longer be a thing. Hopefully, the displaced experts and interlopers will have the capacity and desire to upskill and fill millions of high-value, high-paying jobs in critical fields like cybersecurity, software engineering, etcetera.

It's broadly acknowledged that approximately 25-percent of American health care spending is considered administrative waste. That waste exists primarily because of the fraud and abuse enabled by the idiosyncrasies of fee-for-service transactions. Once vanquished, American health care transactions will be more straightforward, dramatically cheaper to execute, and easier to understand. Rising from the ashes of the vanquished fee-for-service ecosystem will be a fully automated patient-centered approach to health records management, encounter data capture, data analytics, and population-based payment.

Yes. Hospital-centric, Electronic Health Records (EHRs) optimized to facilitate fee-for-service Revenue Cycle Management (RCM) are headed for the trash heap.

Sorry, Judy. No, I'm not sorry.

Your tyrannical reign must end.

DLT will enable fully automated Personal Health Records (PHRs) wholly-owned and fully controlled by the patient. Permissioned access will be granted by patients or those they designate.

Information blocking by payers and providers will be abolished.

It will be technically infeasible.

With automated smart contract protocols enabled by DLT, traditional payers may be joining traditional EHR companies on the trash heap.

3. <u>Federalize the Medicaid program</u>. The federal government finances the vast majority of all Medicaid spending. Majority. Administering dozens of different Medicaid programs is costly and complex.

Complying with different esoteric Medicaid contracting rules is costly, complex, and infuriating for providers. While some providers only operate in one state, many are employed by large health systems functioning across multiple states. The only stakeholders that truly benefit from the Medicaid program's current structure are the American health care cartel and state-focused government contractors.

Weaning them off the gravy train will be challenging.

In addition to the cost and complexities associated with the current design and administration of the Medicaid program, several race-based health disparities are exacerbated because of it.

Every year, many pregnant women and infants rely on Medicaid for health care access.

Particularly low-income Black women and their infants.

Race-based health disparities are exacerbated by partisan decisions of certain states' refusal to expand Medicaid. Other states choose not to offer adequate Medicaid benefits. Market dynamics also come into play. Patients can't benefit from Medicaid coverage if most providers in their community decide not to accept it.

I don't fault the providers, though.

It's not worth the hassle in several states.

Many providers opt to provide charity care instead.

Why stress over crumbs from Medicaid's coffers?

Why bother going through the hassle of Medicaid certification?

Helping to care for the sick and vulnerable is all many providers want to do.

Federalizing Medicaid will simplify American health care by consolidating all programs into a national Medicaid program similar to how the Medicare program is administered. Medicaid Advantage will be established. A national standard-of-care would ensure that everyone enrolled in the Medicaid program has equitable access to health care regardless of which state they choose to live in.

It's sickening that so many Americans silently observe this manner of injustice.

All Americans should have equitable access to federally funded programs they qualify for regardless of which state they live in. Until that ideal scenario is actualized, pro-democracy Americans must flee from states that ruthlessly restrict access to Medicaid.

Federalizing Medicaid will reduce the global cost of administering the program.

It will also provide relief to state budgets.

States will be encouraged to redirect any planned budget outlays for Medicaid towards sustainably developing and scaling local public health infrastructure.

States will be incentivized to allocate planned Medicaid funds towards addressing Social Drivers of Health

(SDoH) and Long Term Services and Supports (LTSS). I can't erase images of hordes of Americans lining up to collect donated food and water during the COVID-19 pandemic. Prosperous nation? Those images suggest otherwise. Unless there's a new definition for the word prosperous that I am not aware of.

A travesty that was unfolding as expensive hospital campuses lay fallow.

Campuses that state budgets had over-allocated resources to construct.

4. <u>Democratize medical education</u>. The Professional Medical Training (PMT) process is currently designed to uphold hospital-centric care. It is very academic. Unbelievably so.

There is a reason the profession is referred to as the practice of medicine.

A reimagined PMT process will be almost entirely practicum or work-studies.

An apprenticeship model in the truest sense of the word.

The reimagined PMT process will establish multiple pathways to achieving physician status. The current PMT process will be enhanced to improve the quality of life of trainees who opt to stick with the status quo.

The vast majority will be trained in a reimagined PMT process.

A reimagined PMT process will introduce significant flexibility. It will encourage individuals going through the process to rotate through all the clinical team roles in their chosen path.

Instead of dedicating 4-years to undergraduate studies

and another 4-years of medical school training, trainees can start receiving medical practicum training immediately after graduating from high school. Exceptional students can start the reimagined PMT process immediately after graduating from middle school.

The mind is a terrible thing to waste, a terrible thing to suppress.

The reimagined model will embrace a hybrid and decentralized team-based approach. Independent physician-led practices, free-standing Ambulatory Surgical Centers (ASCs), and trauma centers will be accredited as practicum and work-study institutions.

I'm not advocating for the elimination of standardized competency assessments. In fact, those competency assessments will carry more weight in the reimagined PMT process.

A trainee that starts as a Medical Assistant with an independent physician-led practice will be incentivized to concurrently pursue self-guided academic learning to round out their knowledge-base. Satisfactorily completing competency assessments would be required to move to the next phase of the reimagined PMT process.

Trainees may choose to terminate or suspend their PMT process at any phase.

Licensure requirements will remain.

A reimagined PMT process would place that Medical Assistant on a career track to complete the Licensed Practical Nurse (LPN) competency assessment. The LPN will be followed by the Registered Nurse (RN) assessment. Attending medical school will be optional in the reimagined PMT process.

Medical College Admission Test (MCATs) will be optional.

Instead of spending years sitting in classrooms and filleting cadavers, trainees will hone their skills by dedicating hours to practicum in their preferred clinical path and team-based learning environment. Enrollment into the medical internship phase would require trainees to successfully complete all existing requirements—step examinations, board examinations, etcetera.

Advanced Practice Professionals (APPs) like Nurse Practitioners (NPs) and Physician Assistants (PA) will be retitled Associate Physician.

Retitling isn't merely a cosmetic change.

It is designed to address condescending patient and physician attitudes towards APPs.

The reimagined PMT process will have a simplified and self-directed career ladder.

1. Medical Assistant.
2. Licensed Practical Nurse.
3. Registered Nurse.
4. Associate Physician.
5. Physician.

That is it. Simple. Straightforward. Scalable.

While the reimagined PMT process is reconstructed with family medicine in mind, the reimagined PMT process can be applied to a range of subspecialties. With time-in-role and competency assessment requirements, trainees will be empowered to pursue the career path that works best for the work-life balance they seek.

No more obscene student loan debt. No more languishing in classrooms consuming esoteric knowledge with no practical application.

No more centralized "gatekeepers."

No more Match Day.

The list goes on.

The reimagined PMT process empowers medical trainees to maximize their potential while helping to address physician shortages in local health markets across the nation. The reimagined PMT process will incentivize medical trainees to enjoy a better quality of life and a balanced existence.

More control over where they work, how much they earn, and how many hours they work.

Implementing a reimagined PMT process will shift some congressionally appropriated Graduate Medical Education (GME) funding from hospital-centric Academic Medical Centers (AMCs) to accredited independent physician-led practices, Ambulatory Surgical Centers (ASCs), and trauma centers.

New authorities and regulations will be required. I'm aware.

5. <u>Incentivize provider independence</u>. The federal government can establish a national medical service workforce of independent providers practicing at the top of their license.

   Abolish state laws that unnecessarily restrict scope of practice. Providers that choose to enroll will also benefit from federal supremacy licensure laws. Participating providers will establish Direct Contracting (DC) relationships with the federal government. Participating providers will receive population-based payment for the lives they manage as Primary Care Providers (PCPs). The federal government will offer simplified outcomes-based bundle payments for specialists that choose to participate in the program. A federally-funded DLT transaction platform will be made available to providers who choose to participate.

Student loans will be forgiven for all participating providers transitioning from being employed by a health system to independent practice. The same offer will be extended to providers that are already practicing independently.

Grants will be made available to finance the transition to independent practice, technical assistance required to support practice administration, and technology adoption for the first 10-years.

In return, each participating PCP will be required to have a patient panel of at least 1,000 patients enrolled in the Medicaid program. Participating PCPs must offer in-home and virtual care modalities, and they must proactively help patients coordinate access to social services.

Medicaid rates for managed lives will be dramatically reduced.

Medicaid value-based bundled payments will have stringent penalties for adverse outcomes.

Wait.

Did you think I would recommend that providers get all that investment and free stuff from the federal government without getting something meaningful back in return?

Ah!

I'm not that guy.

I'm truly in it to accrue benefits to patients and taxpayers.

That's it.

6. <u>Modernize and integrate federal innovation efforts</u>. The White House must establish a Federal Innovation Council led by a Federal Chief Innovation Officer (CINO) that reports directly to the OMB Director.

   The Federal CINO will collaborate with the Federal Chief Information Officer (CIO) and Directors of the White House Domestic Policy Council (DPC) and the White House National Economic Council (NEC).

   Collectively, they will design and implement a comprehensive strategy to reimagine how the federal government functions.

   They will chart a more prosperous path for America.

   The Federal CINO will have the Principal Associate Directors (PADs) for Health and National Security as direct reports. This reporting structure will ensure there is a dedicated and knowledgeable voice advocating for effective health reform policy near the top of the OMB reporting structure. Always.

   The PAD for Health oversees federal payer and provider assets administered by the Department of Health and Human Services (HHS).

   The PAD for National Security oversees federal payer and provider assets administered by the Department of Veterans Affairs (VA) and the Defense Health Agency (DHA).

   Political appointees serving in both PAD roles and the career civil servants that report to them have limited insight into the rules and authorities of the other groups' portfolio of programs. They have a limited understanding of opportunities to integrate innovation efforts across the two portfolios.

Very few people can recognize and implement opportunities to leverage authorities and assets administered by HHS, VA, and DHA. Opportunities to dramatically transform American health care delivery and payments.

The Federal Health System directs 35-percent of national health spending.

Taxpayers should be getting more bang for our buck.

Instead, we are being exploited.

American prosperity, decaying.

The federal share of national health spending is expected to grow exponentially in the next decade and beyond.

The Federal CINO will be empowered to integrate health innovation efforts across HHS, VA, and DHA. Such integration will empower the three groups to maximize their collective innovation potential.

The Federal CINO will collaborate with the CMS Administrator to coordinate value-based care initiatives across the Federal Health System. There's more to it than just Medicare and Medicaid. Other programs in the Federal Health portfolio include; Veterans Health Administration (VHA), Defense Health Administration (DHA), Indian Health Service (IHS), Federal Employee Health Benefits (FEHB), and the Federal Bureau of Prisons (BOP).

Federal inmates receive health care.

At least they are supposed to.

The Federal CINO will collaborate with Congress to establish a reimagined Chief Innovation Officer (CINO) role and office of innovation at all Federal Agencies. The reimagined offices of innovation will be designed to function as the carrot to the Office of Inspector General's stick.

CINOs will be endowed with authorities and resources similar to the Inspector General appointed to each agency. CINOs will have the autonomy and resources required to reimagine and pilot innovative operating models for their respective agencies.

Innovative models designed to effectively meet their mission. Now and in the future.

7. <u>Establish a federal virtual health care delivery system with federal supremacy</u>. The Federal Innovation Council can coordinate the development and scaling of a publicly-run virtual health care delivery system. A Distributed Ledger Technology (DLT) platform optimized to facilitate on-demand and scheduled virtual visits to all members of the American population. Even when they are overseas.

Hundreds of thousands of Americans were stuck overseas when COVID-19 travel bans were first instituted.

Some were stuck for months.

Some suffered needlessly.

Some died without access to health care.

Americans.

Taxpayers.

Our sons and daughters.

Our brothers and sisters.

Our mothers and fathers.

We _can_ do better.

We _must_ do better.

We _will_ do better.

The virtual health care delivery system must be powered by DLT architecture. Value-based incentives and payment models will be embedded in smart contract protocols that enable seamless, secure, low-cost transactions between all users.

The Federal Innovation Council and participating agency CINOs will enable the virtual health care delivery system's ongoing operations and management. While the DLT platform would be publicly run, the providers and patients that utilize the platform will wholly own and permission any user-generated data. The government will pay participating providers based on the lowest negotiated federal reimbursement rate for any covered beneficiary. Private payers will reimburse at negotiated rates.

Licensed and accredited providers and producers based in America will have the autonomy to set market-clearing prices below negotiated rates. Dynamic pricing capabilities will be programmable into the DLT platform. However, providers and producers will be unable to offer prices above negotiated rates for covered beneficiaries.

Surge pricing will be permitted for users that aren't covered beneficiaries. Foreigners.

Providers and producers can maintain verified credentials on the DLT platform.

Verified credentials will be seamlessly transmitted across all government platforms.

Federal. State. Local.

Verified credentials will reduce documentation requirements and inefficiencies associated with provider and producer credentialing or certification.

Patients will have the autonomy to select providers and establish recurring subscription agreements. Value-based bundled payment arrangements. Simplified, affordable, and accessible contracts with providers and producers using the virtual health care delivery platform.

The virtual health care delivery platform will enable enhanced and equitable access to clinical trials. Biobank and trial matching features will be integrated.

Patients will receive hospital-level care at home, with remote monitoring.

Veterans Health Administration (VHA) and Indian Health Service (IHS) medical facilities will serve as in-person delivery centers of last resort.

Although competitive, reasonably priced private markets are anticipated, it's always prudent to have a backup.

VHA and IHS would continue to prioritize their respective missions.

Besides, especially with VHA, America's population of veterans is projected to reduce by approximately 30-percent in the next 27-years. According to the Department of Veterans Affairs (VA), the total veteran population is expected to decline from 19.5 million in 2020 to 13.6 million in 2048. VA only provides health care to a third of all veterans. Thankfully, VA provides broader mental health coverage.

Capacity constraints shouldn't be a problem.

The future of American health care will be focused on eliminating unnecessary visits to hospitals and emergency rooms. Chronically ill patients must be kept far away from hospital-centric health system campuses.

They must be kept healthy at home.

The future is consumer-centric care at home.

Care at higher-value, community-based sites of care.

To realize this future and much more, we must reimagine American health care delivery and payments. A reimagined American health care ecosystem will meaningfully leverage technology to reduce health spending while improving health outcomes, equity, access, quality, and experience.

That is a tall order. I am aware.

We need better leaders to establish a reimagined American health care ecosystem.

Better leaders that can rise to the occasion.

Better leaders that can prevent looming and ongoing challenges from becoming calamities Americans suffer through needlessly.

Better leaders will be bolstered by political infrastructure that isn't designed to undermine American prosperity.

As I finish writing this book, I feel a slight sense of relief and hope.

Relief and hope because even though George Floyd's name and character were dragged through the mud during the trial of the White "dude" who murdered him, Americans in the jury held the murderer accountable. Americans found the murderer guilty of all charges. Although slightly relieved, I'm still wary of how light the murderous White "dude's" prison sentence may end up being. I also wonder if his conviction will be overturned on appeal.

Many Americans were mortified by the torture and humiliation George Floyd endured in his final moments. Most Americans don't want to raise our families in a society where unjustified state-sanctioned murders go unpunished. Most Americans are justified in celebrating the conviction of a murderer.

A murderer that was operating as an agent of the state when he committed his heinous crime.

Unfortunately, murderous American police aren't convicted of any crimes 99-percent of the times they unjustifiably murder members of the American population.

Most Americans felt like the conviction of the White "dude" who murdered George Floyd <u>signaled the beginning of a new era in America</u>.

An era of accountability for protected classes of Americans.

Protected classes of Americans that have been operating above the law for centuries.

Fingers crossed.

Although I felt a slight sense of relief after the verdict came in, I remain disturbed as news of senseless mass murders and cases of police brutality continue to be reported.

Almost daily.

These types of violent American deaths left our collective consciousness while thousands of Americans were dying from COVID-19.

Daily.

Thanks to the tireless efforts of the Biden Administration, more than 100 million Americans were fully vaccinated by the end of April 2021.

Unfortunately, many Americans remain skeptical about getting vaccinated. It's unclear if America will ever achieve herd immunity. I assume additional strains of COVID-19 will emerge every year. Heck, we might be dealing with another outbreak and other lockdowns this fall.

COVID-19 is probably here to stay. Endemic.

The question remains: How many Americans will die from new strains of COVID-19 annually?

Though hopeful, I remain perplexed by a lingering question: Will post-pandemic America be better or worse than pre-pandemic America?

Equally concerning are the lasting impacts of long-COVID.

Rising rates of long-COVID diagnosis will join the growing list of trends that will increase the demand on the American health care ecosystem. This increased demand occurs as American health care continues its death march towards increased complexity, spending, and inequities.

Absent any paradigm-shifting interventions, the American health care death march will destroy American prosperity. It will increase American suffering.

I am closing out this book with a somewhat unsettled tone regarding the future.

I am aware. Sad. Frustrated.

Yet, I have faith in humanity.

Faith because I know that <u>the power to enable a better future is within each of us</u>.

There's no time like the present to invent the future we seek.

We shouldn't grow weary in well-doing.

It is up to us to make America what we need it to be.

What our children need it to be.

What the world needs it to be.

We just have to <u>muster the courage to do the right thing</u>.

So, do the right thing.

<u>Organize</u>. <u>Mobilize</u>. <u>Migrate</u>. <u>VOTE</u>!

"The key to realizing a dream is to focus not on success but on significance – and then even the small steps and little victories along your path will take on greater meaning." – Oprah Winfrey

"You don't make progress by standing on the sidelines whimpering and complaining. You make progress by implementing ideas."
– Rep. Shirley Chisholm

"We do not want our freedom gradually, we want to be free now!"

– Rep. John Lewis

Epilogue: Frustrations

"With so many unresolved problems, I don't understand the utility in any society choosing to waste the human potential of its population."

Embracing my Lewis Black mindset...

1. **The most annoying White supremacists.** The most annoying ones are the ones who choose to highlight Black-on-Black homicide whenever there is civil unrest following an unjustified state-sanctioned murder of another Black person by police. The American ritual of the state-sanctioned murder of Black people originated in slavery. This barbaric act continued with establishing the Ku Klux Klan, lynching, and modern-day police brutality. Each iteration and incident is an act of terrorism. An act of terrorism that reminds every Black person that our tax dollars are financing the unjustified state-sanctioned murder of people that look like us. Unjustified state-sanctioned murders remind us that these taxpayer-funded murderers will likely never be held accountable. The morally reprehensible hacks that choose to highlight Black-on-Black homicide after another unjustified state-sanctioned murder by police should consider two things. One, continued propagation of White supremacy by American institutions is the root cause of the ills in Black communities, leading to the disproportionately higher rates of Black-on-Black homicides. Second, police brutality is an act of terrorism.

Expecting the majority of the Black community to focus on the higher numbers of Black-on-Black homicide after another unjustified state-sanctioned murder is akin to the rest of the world expecting America to focus on addressing the more than 13,000 homicides of Americans by other Americans in 2001. After all, the terrorist attacks on September 11, 2001 (9/11) "only" resulted in the killing of fewer than 3,000 Americans on 9/11. No one in their right mind would expect that. Exactly. Beyond a history rooted in slavery, unjustified state-sanctioned murders of Black people by primarily White police officers differ from any other type of murder or violent crime in American society. It is a state-sanctioned act of terrorism. A state that is supposed to protect and defend all Americans. A state that is supposed to uphold the ideals of democracy. It remains a triggering event for most Black people. A triggering event that often reminds every Black person they might be next. Someone they love might be next. A triggering event that reminds most Black people that we are yet to achieve equal protection under the law. **Yuuuuuuuuuuck!**

2. **I'm grateful for America, but I want more.** I'll be the first to acknowledge that America offers more opportunities to marginalized Black people than any other country in the world. However, White supremacists who tell Black people to "get over" slavery and systemic racism by spewing that fact should realize that while those are the facts, those facts don't negate the debilitating impact systemic racism can have on individual families and communities. Individuals, families, and communities that aren't able to cope with racial trauma. Systemic racism is similar to domestic abuse and related trauma. It is diabolical to tell victims of ongoing abuse to stop complaining because their

partner only assaults them when they are drunk or having a bad day. No single incidence should be normalized and considered acceptable. It should never happen. Never. And when it does, we should be willing to punish the abuser with the total weight of the law, especially when the state sponsors the abuser. It is the only decent thing to do. The right thing to do. Victim shaming and victim-blaming are never appropriate. Never. **Yuck!**

3. **Ultra-woke members of the Liberal Left.** They are intentionally absurdifying (Yes, it is a made-up word. Thanks for the inspiration, Dave) inclusion efforts in a sinister attempt to contaminate all Diversity, Equity, and Inclusion (DEI) efforts. Elitist White supremacy™ at work. I wonder if regular woke people will rise to the occasion, call this tactic out, and squash it. Inequities aren't equal. Inequities that persist because American institutions propagate White supremacy are very different from perceived inequities that exist from the use of the gender-associated label "mother." I remain appalled that there is a growing push to mainstream the use of "birthing people" instead of mothers. I mean, come on. Seriously? Inequities caused by race, gender, and sexual orientation are in a different category from all the other inequities the ultra-woke crowd is harping on. Conflating the two groups of inequities is a dangerous, blatant, and offensive attempt to contaminate higher priority inequities that shouldn't have to share the stage or limelight with preposterous nonsense like the "birthing people" debate. Mothers and fathers can both be nurturing. Providing direct care and affection to children males and females help create and raise shouldn't be restricted to the person in the role of the mother. The notion that our parental nomenclature should be updated to include "birthing

people" is merely a symptom of widespread undiagnosed mental illness and unresolved sexual trauma in the population of the ultra-woke hacks advocating for this change. Yes, they are elitist White supremacists. White supremacy is a form of delusional thinking. Delusional thinking is a severe mental illness. White supremacy is a severe mental illness. A severe mental illness characterized by unshakable beliefs in things that aren't true or rooted in reality. **Yuuuuuck!**

4. **Racists who consider themselves followers of Jesus Christ.** Racists have no understanding of the Jesus they claim to be serving or following. Yes, I said it. I don't understand the cognitive dissonance that is pervasive across the White evangelical community. How can someone claim to follow Jesus and despise his children? Claim to love a god they've never seen but are quick to oppress and desecrate his creations? What kind of love is that? That is not loving. Not even close. There's nothing spiritual or godly about racist people. Nothing. Yes. I'm judging. I'm allowed. Racists are liars and hypocrites who try to hide behind the bible—hiding from the truth and trying to replicate the evil of their ancestors who used the bible to subjugate my ancestors. They are trying to use the bible to silence the oppressed masses in America. Stop preaching. Do the work. Come and join us in our fight for justice. Be on the right side of history. Seek peace, love, and fairness. Jesus is Lord.

5. **Military veterans and physicians are committing suicide at alarming rates.** What kind of a society are we living in here in America? People working in the noblest professions are the ones killing themselves at the highest rates? And we are ok with that? I suspect hopelessness and higher rates of exposure to trauma

are causing some of it. Why are they hopeless, you ask? Physicians have elevated exposure to trauma and stress. More work is being piled on them as the American health care cartel makes more money off the bloated health care ecosystem. Military veterans have exposure to trauma and stress. They have strained family relationships. Exposure to significant amounts of physical and emotional trauma. Loss of a sense of purpose after transitioning to civilian life. Loss of meaning and fulfillment in work after transitioning to civilian life and going from leading dozens, hundreds, thousands, or more in defense of America to pushing paper in civilian life. Often dealing with toxic corporate cultures. Loss of good pay in certain instances. I don't have any answers. I just hate the fact that so many veterans and physicians are killing themselves. We are aware of the problem. We are aware of some of the root causes. Will America ever wake up and do the right thing? On this severe issue? And others? **Yuuuuuuuuuuck!**

6. **America's self-defeating strategy.** White mediocrity is rapidly decaying American society into a North American version of Brazil. It's so blatant. It's disgusting. Yes. Being enslaved in Brazil during the Trans-Atlantic slave trade was much worse than being enslaved in America. Yes. Being Black in Brazil today is much worse than being Black in America. I am aware. I am grateful. Brazil isn't unique. America can devolve into Brazil. The outcomes we achieve are a direct result of the actions we take. Magical creatures don't live in America. We are all human. Trump and his team were probably taking pointers from Bolsonaro and his team. Fascists can't be elevated to the highest offices ever again. Never again. American democracy will not survive it. Western democracy won't survive it. American democracy needs

to be strengthened, not weakened. For the knuckle-dragging purists, Argentinian history with the Trans-Atlantic slave trade and post-abolition genocide is a manifestation of the wildest dreams of American White supremacists. Present-day Argentina is 97-percent "White." The Argentinian economy and society still suck for the hordes of "White people" that live there. I wish more people would embrace an equitable American democracy. The world needs America to maximize its potential. **Yuuuuuuuuuuck!**

7. **Perils of Whitewashing.** Bribery is a crime, but lobbying is legal? Seriously? Utter nonsense. The ultimate manifestation of the insidious Whitewashing of criminal behavior. The audacity of White supremacy never ceases to amaze me. As if people don't have common sense. Something is wrong. Harmful. Insidious. And yet, they want us to pretend as if there is some logical reason why lobbying should be allowed. Some logical reason why we should accept that regular Americans will just continue to take the abuse and exploitation forever. They should rue the day the oppressed masses unite and call horse manure on all the different ways they have artificially divided us. Whitewashing is so toxic. It's so frustrating. It's so damaging. I don't know why some of these practices continue. I mean. Everyone read The Emperor's New Clothes. At least when I was growing up. And Animal Farm. This kind of behavior doesn't end well. It doesn't. **Yuuuuuuuuuuck!**

8. **Why continue the American tradition of hyphenation?** It artificially divides the masses. The words we use matter. Granted, naturalized citizens still have their country of birth listed in their American passports. Still. Why do so many Americans want to keep this practice going? Folks who were born here or folks who adopted

America as their home. We are better together. We are stronger together. We are more interesting together. We should all embrace the same identifiers. American. Sure, folks can list their ancestry afterward. Maybe also throw in race afterward. It shouldn't be such a controversial point of view. Especially if it helps bridge any gaps or divides. Yes, the White people started it so everyone else could have a constant reminder that they could get sent back to where they once came. Yes, I've had several iterations of "go back to Africa" thrown in my face. All American imports came from somewhere. We aren't going anywhere. Let's make it work here. Let's make it work, so our children don't have to deal with this mess. I am an American man of Nigerian ancestry. Christian. Melanated. Pragmatist. Maximizer.

9. **Rich people are parking their philanthropic dollars.** Wasted money is an unbelievably frustrating thing to witness. I'm not even so sure at this point if it matters how the money-wasting is happening. It isn't achieving the stated goals. Then it is wasted. Parking in a Donor-Advised-Fund (DAF)? No impact. Why make public announcements expressing a desire to achieve impact when the impact never materializes? Year after year. Decade after decade. No results. No impact. Pontificating viewpoints with no implementation strategy, just talking about infeasible things, wishfully thinking. The whole lot should admit they were wrong and direct their resources toward the only thing that can make any other reform they pursuing realize any meaningful impact. Campaign finance reform helps address partisan gerrymandering and voter suppression laws. If we get rid of all three, we have a chance to improve American institutions and American democracy. That's it. That's the shot—that where the impact is. Everything else is just a waste of time. Why

endure another decade of mediocre results? C'mon. Get in the actual game. **Yuck!**

10. **Intelligent people are committing to low-impact careers.** My rational mind gets it. Most people are financially constrained or resigned to the fact that most things won't move the needle. They won't. Based on that reality, I get why many folks don't care what they do for a living. As long as it's something they are competent at and pays the bills, they are all for it. The reality still frustrates me, though. Especially the luminaries. I mean. These are supposed to be the smartest people in the room and are constantly getting outsmarted by random cartel guys whose overwhelming strategy is to become a monopoly? The only game they can win is the one where they are the only ones playing? Those guys? It's like you think we were born yesterday. If you are the smartest person in the room and you are getting outsmarted all the time, leave the room. Let someone else be the smartest person in the room. Or maybe the truth is that these "luminaries" are merely Low Impact Experts (LIEs). Apt. **Yuck!**

11. **Why aren't Incumbents called out for faking it?** Am I the only one paying attention to what Ascension is doing? They made the song and dance on the high-volume Centers of Excellence strategy. Even combined it with medical tourism. Even entered into a Joint Venture Agreement with Narayana Health to establish Health City Cayman Islands (HCCI). Per usual. It was just a ruse. They eventually pulled out and went back to their bread and butter. Hospital-centric care. **Yuck!** Home health is the new frontier they supposedly care about improving. I assume the outcome will be the same. They influence policy and regulations to favor

hospitals and create dependencies with partners in the home health coalition. Partners they will leave high and dry when it suits them. So annoying. Mayo Clinic and Humana are flinging the same shtick about home health. This strategy makes sense for Humana as a payer. It doesn't make as much sense for Mayo Clinic. Only time will tell. I'm watching the space. I hope I'm wrong about why Ascension and Mayo Clinic are involved. It's so hard for incumbents to change, though. **Yuuuuuck!**

12. **Will anything stop the monopolistic ambitions of UnitedHealth Group?** I'm pretty sure I'm not the only one seeing this. Like a slow-moving train that will eventually arrive at its intended destination, UnitedHealth Group is slowly moving towards world domination. Andrew Witty is now CEO. I assume they want to go after NHS contracts. I wish the U.K. good luck. I hope it works out for them. I would advise lawyers at UnitedHealth Group to examine European Union anti-cartel regulations. If UnitedHealth Group takes certain practices across the pond, it could be their undoing. There is nothing inherently evil about UnitedHealth Group. I don't like incumbents that much because they don't ever really deliver paradigm-shifting change. They jettison anything disruptive, innovative, and paradigm-shifting. They keep armies of people on staff who would otherwise become the entrepreneurs that build companies that replace theirs. I met with senior executives at UnitedHealth Group back in 2019. Dirk McMahon, the President and COO of UnitedHealth Group, and Patty Horoho, the CEO of OptumServe, were the two most senior executives from the UnitedHealth Group team that attended that meeting. I think they had 15 other folks in the room. I lost count. There were only 6 or so folks from VA in attendance. I requested the

meeting. I was hoping to chart a seismic collaborative vision to transform American health care.

It didn't pan out. I wanted to hear from the horse's mouth if UnitedHealth Group intended to do anything transformational. They talked about RallyHealth, Big Data, NPS scores. Blah-blah. That didn't do it for me. The monopoly strategy is pretty lame. Sheesh! I had a table-pounding moment before they confirmed they weren't building an alternative to fee-for-service architecture. I was visibly irritated when Dirk finally owned up to this fact. If UnitedHealth Group isn't making that shift, none of the incumbents are. That means the industry is committed to fee-for-service. That sucks. We need a law abolishing fee-for-service transactions. It is never going to evolve into an effective value-based platform. It just won't. I also tried working with the OptumServe team on a new, paradigm-shifting approach to bundled payments. Feedback: It is too innovative. Typical. **Yuck!**

13. **Winning strategy for data aggregators?** The primary data aggregators will be an interesting bunch to watch. I think Google comes out ahead since they are primarily supporting the American health care cartel. Amazon is competing with a toe-dipping strategy that will likely backfire. In any event, these data aggregators want more information to help their algorithms and advertisement sales. That is it. They are just pushing folks to expand their data, compute, and storage needs by any means necessary. The end game doesn't make any sense. Yeah, it's good to have cloud storage, data analytics, etcetera. To what end? They want to aggregate data. They want to store information. Ok. How does that improve health care in a meaningful way? It doesn't even save money. Big Data and biased algorithms will only lead to more misdiagnosis and

wasteful spending. Just like the American health care cartel ordered.

Nothing has improved quality, so I'm not even going to bother with that one. This strategy is just moving bloated expenses from some health system fat and converting it into Google Cloud and analytics revenue. But hey. They have the stuff to sell, and they convinced someone to buy. Let's all stop pretending like Big Data is some panacea. It isn't. Medical services only account for 10-percent of what helps people achieve good health outcomes. 10-percent. That is all. If Google Health and Google Cloud want to be innovative, they should figure out how to leverage their assets to improve factors that account for 90-percent of what keeps people healthy. They could even explore things that have nothing to do with training their advertising algorithms.

Unfortunately, money and profits always win those battles. Godspeed Karen. I'm not holding my breath. Amazon, with its Amazon Care ambitions, will have to decide at some point. Is the mighty AWS business on the chopping block? I know it's not. So why piss off the American health care cartel with the Amazon Care thing? Or the pharma ambitions? If the American health care cartel gets pissed off enough at Amazon Care, they will activate their membership to start canceling their AWS contracts. Andy Jassy is now Amazon CEO. He's not going to let anything happen to AWS. His baby. Health care isn't like anything else. Casual encounters leave most with STDs. Even committed relationships can result in significant abuse. Unless the American health care cartel is dismantled, new entrants will either play by cartel rules or get squashed. Those are the two choices. There's no "winning." New entrants have to make it their primary focus to have a shot at staying in the game. Otherwise, it unlikely they will survive for long. **Yuck!**

14. **HCAPHS Paper Surveys. Still? Seriously?** The Hospital Consumer Assessment of Healthcare Providers and Systems (HCAPHS) is still primarily paper-based. Just so that the U.S. Postal Service will have some additional volume. Same thing with mail-in-ballots. Must everything be a jobs program? Maybe USPS deliveries should only happen once a week. Let FedEx, UPS, Amazon, and Walmart handle expedited shipping and mailing. Alternatively, if we must have daily USPS mail delivery, we could convert USPS into a federal PBM delivery arm or visiting nurses. USPS leaders need to be creative.

    Not having a centralized digital standard for patient experience encounter data capture is very annoying and inefficient. Very. But because there are so many human jobs supporting the current inefficient process, the powers that be don't want to mess with it. Most people wouldn't ordinarily care, but HCAPHS scores are among the items they include in most hospital STAR ratings. It is a measure of quality. So people are mailing forms. People are filling those forms. People are sending the papers back. People are sorting through those forms to organize for intake. People are entering data into a computer. If HCAPHS were digital, USPS could automate the manual workflows; all the mailing activities would be gone. So would the jobs. I wonder if the powers that be realize that being stuck in a mind-numbing career when millions of higher-value, higher-skilled jobs go unfilled is a terrible outcome for any society. USPS is the second-largest civilian employer in America. The second-largest! Sheesh! Trillions of brain cells dying every day as their human hosts primarily deliver junk mail and move through the same mail routes like hamsters on a wheel. **Yuck!**

15. **Whoosah.** I could go on. But I think you get the point...We have a lot of work to do. **Yuck!**

"To thrive, societies must prioritize nurturing talent and enabling the highest and best use of everyone's time and energy."

"This is no time to engage in the luxury of cooling off or to take the tranquilizing drug of gradualism.

*Now is the time to make real
the promises of democracy.*

*Now is the time to rise from the dark and desolate valley of segregation to the sunlit path
of racial justice.*

*Now is the time... to lift our nation from the quicksand's of racial injustice
to the solid rock of brotherhood.*

*Now is the time to make justice a reality
for all of God's children."*

– Dr. Martin Luther King Jr.
From Dr. King's historic "I Have a Dream" speech
during the 1963 March on Washington.

Acknowledgments

"Why tip-toe through life to arrive safely at death?"
– Christopher 'Ludacris' Bridges

First and foremost, I'd like to thank my Lord and Savior Jesus Christ for blessing me with a community of family and friends who keep me grounded and challenge me to be a better person. I give honor to my late father, Professor Isaac Olaoluwa Akinyele. His untimely, sudden death in 2014 ignited my desire to help catalyze the creation of an affordable and accessible global health care system.

I would like to thank my exceptional and gorgeous wife, Bolanle, and our amazing children. I appreciated their patience and consideration as I organized my thoughts, put pen to paper, and wrote this book. Their unconditional love, compassion, character, and devotion to the success of our family inspire and challenge me to be a better man, husband, and father.

I am eternally grateful to God that they are an integral part of my life and legacy. I love each of them with every fiber of my being. I pray to God every day that I have the years, patience, and capacity to support their life ambitions as they maximize their potential.

I would like to thank my dear mother, Professor Ayoni Faderera Akinyele. I'm eternally grateful for her unconditional love, faith in Christ, passion for my book☺, patience, wisdom, character, and her undying support and sacrifice for the success of my nuclear family. I'm thankful she could share her childhood stories and feedback throughout my process of writing this book. I'm eternally grateful that she is continuing the oral tradition of passing down wisdom to the next generation, sharing her experiences growing up in Ejigbo, and marrying into the Akinyele family.

This book involved the behind-the-scenes contributions of many people, to which I am forever indebted. My supportive, thoughtful, and diverse village of copy editors challenged me to simplify, crystalize, and breathe life into my words. I owe you☺. The guidance and insight I received as I iterated on different drafts of this book were essential to framing my writing style, the structure, and the sequencing of the various chapters.

I'm grateful for two of my sisters. I love all my siblings but only asked two to help copy-edit my book. Alice, born a year before me. A Howard alumna who went on to earn her Juris Doctorate from Georgetown University. Deborah, born a year after me. A Howard alumna who went on to earn a Master's degree from George Washington University and is working on her Doctorate. They have known me my entire life. They watched me grow up. They acknowledged I was in rare form with this book. Ha-ha. I appreciate their insightful feedback on the earliest versions of this book and my natural writing style. Addressing the gaps they highlighted in my earliest drafts enabled me to improve my approach to writing the initial drafts of the later chapters. I'm grateful they helped me refine my voice and tone. They were curtailing my gratuitous use of incendiary language. Yeah. This version of the book is edgy but filtered. Maybe I need to write an unfiltered version. Maybe.

I'm thankful for my favorite American dad, Dave Burris. He is an American man of European ancestry who happens to be Melanemic (humans with low ratios of eumelanin in their skin), Agnostic, and progressive. He retired from the Internal Revenue Service (IRS) after 25-years as a Special Agent in the Criminal Division. He also earned a Master's in Public Health (MPH). As our relationship enters its sixteenth year, I'm eternally grateful that we were paired together in 2006, and he became my career counselor. I'm thankful for his wisdom, support, wit, love, and guidance over the years. I appreciate his thoughtful, critical, and valuable feedback as I wrote and published this book.

I'm forever indebted to my dear friends (some who will remain anonymous☺) who helped me organize my thinking on the structure, design, themes, and tone of my book while contributing thoughtfully to my work in immeasurable ways. As the Bible says in Proverbs Chapter 11 verse 14, wisdom emerges in the multitude of counsel.

I want to thank my Stanford Graduate School of Business (GSB) class of 2012 crew of copy editors. I'm grateful for the depth of perspective they shared and for challenging me not to rely entirely on my intuition when writing this book. I remain eternally thankful for their valuable contributions and for allowing me to learn from their experiences.

Grateful for Onuche 'Onu' Ocholi, an American man of Nigerian ancestry who happens to be Melanated (humans with high ratios of eumelanin in their skin) and Christian. Currently residing in the U.K., he and I lived in the same Munger residential building during our first year at the GSB. I appreciate the brutal honesty in his feedback regarding the structure of the initial chapters and the original sequence of this book. The first draft was an absolute mess☺. The additional nuggets of wisdom he shared were precious. The nuggets of wisdom he shared helped me look at certain aspects of this book in slightly different but meaningfully impactful ways.

Grateful for Fareeda Ahmed, an American woman of South-Asian ancestry who happens to be Melanated, Muslim and progressive. She also lived in the same Munger residential building as Onu and me during our first year at the GSB. I'm thankful for her guidance, which helped me see the wisdom of simplifying each chapter's central argument. I'm also grateful for her encouragement, especially as it pertains to getting the themes I share in this book out into the world.

Grateful for Joe Dimento, an American man of European ancestry who happens to be Melanemic, Atheist and progressive. I enjoyed sharing countless hours with Joe during our GSB Interpersonal Dynamics (Touchy-Feely) classes, T-Group sessions, and the T-Group weekend retreat. I'm thankful for his invaluable insights and keen eye. Those keen insights helped shape the structure and sequencing of this book. The thoughtfulness and depth of his feedback challenged my thinking, as always.

Grateful for Mary Ellen Richardson Player (MERP), an American woman of European ancestry who happens to be Melanemic, Christian, and progressive. She's an antiracist southern belle. I enjoyed getting to know MERP during the planning and execution of the 2012 student-led GER trip to Nigeria and Ghana that she co-led. With my book, I'm thankful for her immeasurable and precise contributions. Despite the tight deadline, she rose to the occasion and shared valuable insights as usual.

I would also like to thank my International School of Ibadan (ISI) class of 2000 classmates who contributed to copy-editing, Yoruba tone mark validation, translation of proverbs, and book cover design. I appreciate their responsiveness and support given the compressed timelines I put them under☺. I'm eternally grateful for their friendship.

Grateful for Oyeleke Alabi, a Nigerian man and U.K. resident who grew up in Ibadan and is Melanated, Christian, and conservative. A dear friend from Junior Secondary School (JSS) 1B I met during our first term at ISI more than 25-years ago. *We don old o.* I am thankful he remained a steward of the Yoruba language. He helped validate our shared cultural history represented in this book. I'm also grateful he helped me verify the appropriate tone marks on the many Yoruba words I included in this book.

Grateful for Adeyokunnu 'Adey' Adedayo, a Nigerian man from Osun state who happens to be Melanated, Christian, and progressive. He currently splits his time between the U.K. and Nigeria. I didn't interact with Adey much when we were at ISI. I wasn't part of the "in-crowd." He was one of the "cool guys" and rumored to be much older than the rest of us in our set. He isn't. It turns out I'm older than him. I've gotten to know him pretty well since. We have had several lengthy debates on far-ranging topics. He has a passion for arguing. Is it your father's business? Thankful he added his creative vision to the design of my book cover. He also passionately encouraged me to publish this book. While I consider Adey an intelligent and rational human being, I'll never understand why he is a fervent and vocal supporter of President Buhari. I guess his passions consume him from time to time and prevent him from seeing reason.

I am grateful for my cousin, Adefolaju 'Fola' Tella, a Nigerian man residing in Lagos who happens to be Melanated, Christian, and progressive. I appreciate his creative genius and critical feedback as I evolved my book's cover design. Even though he represented Nigeria in the Cannes festival (Young Lion Print and Ad category 2015 and 2016), I'm glad he agreed to collaborate on this effort even though I told him that I would retain veto power on the final cover design. I will gladly let him actualize his vision for the second print edition. Assuming there is a second print☺.

Last but not least, I would like to express my profound gratitude to my namesake and brother from another mother, Professor Michael Esman Chernew. He is an American man of Jewish ancestry who happens to be Melanemic and centrist. He is easily my favorite health economist since his horse manure meter is almost as strong as mine. He is similarly wary of health reform snake oil and authentic in assessing the potential impact of health reform proposals. I'm thankful for the many health policy debates we've had over the years and our shared frustration with where America is in its health reform journey.

Thankful he shared his wisdom and incredibly grateful he agreed to write the foreword to my debut book. I hope he doesn't get any blowback. Fingers crossed. I appreciate his attempts (some were successful) to dissuade me from gratuitously using language some may consider inflammatory and likely turn off fragile readers. If this version of the book gets traction, I'll plan to publish alternate versions that probably appeal to a broader audience. Despite all that, I'm comfortable leading with this version of the book. Even if it's the only one I ever get to write.

Finally, for everyone who took the time to read my book, I'm grateful you took a chance on my debut book. I know you had many other ways you could've spent your time, so I'm thankful you took the time to read my book. I hope you were enlightened and found the content valuable.

"A positive mind finds a way it can be done;
a negative mind looks for all the ways it can't be done."
– Napoleon Hill

About the Author

"Anyone can add value. But if you judge a lion on its ability to sing, it will assume its roar is worthless."

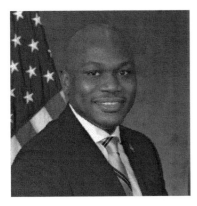

Michael Akinyele is the Founder and Managing Principal of The Maximizer Group, a startup venture studio and independent advisory firm primarily advising startup companies, investors, and corporations. He is a collaborative leader, product and growth expert, and a health care futurist focused on inventing the future of health care delivery and payments.

He is the former Founding Chief Innovation Officer of the U.S. Department of Veterans Affairs (VA), the largest federal civilian agency with an annual budget greater than $250 billion and more than 400 thousand employees. He was appointed to the Senior Executive Service (SES) in 2019 and was responsible for leading, transforming, and scaling enterprise innovation at VA.

He primarily focused on implementing Section 152 of the MISSION Act of 2018, which authorized the creation of a Center for Innovation for Care and Payment at the VA. He was the Principal Lead of the VA Innovation Center (VIC) and served in that capacity from March 2018 to September 2020. Before his work at the VA, his most recent full-time role was serving as the Director of Venture Development — Health Care at a private foundation with approximately $2 billion in assets and more than $100 million in annual disbursements.

Before his role in philanthropy, he led management consulting teams focused on developing and implementing solutions to strategic and operational challenges facing multinational corporations. He has advised health systems, physician groups, academic medical centers, health plans, pharmaceutical companies, pharmacy benefit managers, and a Medicaid agency in the American health care industry.

He is a member of for-profit and non-profit boards and is concurrently incubating and launching several new ventures designed to reinvent the American health care system.

Mr. Akinyele started his career managing physician practices in the Washington, D.C. metro area. He earned his Master's in Business Administration from Stanford Graduate School of Business and graduated magna cum laude with a bachelor's degree in Economics from Howard University.

Follow @MOAkinyele | References, visit www.themaximizergroup.com

Join the discussion at https://michaeloakinyele.substack.com/

To stay up to date with the authors work and learn about future events, subscribe to our newsletter at https://themaximizergroup.com/engage/

Made in the USA
Las Vegas, NV
17 June 2021